RELIGION AND HEALTH CARE IN EAST AFRICA

Lessons from Uganda, Mozambique and Ethiopia

Robert B. Lloyd, Melissa Haussman
and Patrick James

First published in Great Britain in 2019 by Policy Press an Imprint of Bristol University Press

Policy Press
University of Bristol
1-9 Old Park Hill
Bristol
BS2 8BB
UK
t: +44 (0)117 954 5940
pp-info@bristol.ac.uk
www.policypress.co.uk

North America office:
Policy Press
c/o The University of Chicago Press
1427 East 60th Street
Chicago, IL 60637, USA
t: +1 773 702 7700
f: +1 773-702-9756
sales@press.uchicago.edu
www.press.uchicago.edu

© Policy Press 2019

British Library Cataloguing in Publication Data
A catalogue record for this book is available from the British Library

Library of Congress Cataloging-in-Publication Data
A catalog record for this book has been requested

ISBN 978-1-4473-3787-4 hardcover
ISBN 978-1-4473-3789-8 ePub
ISBN 978-1-4473-3800-0 Mobi
ISBN 978-1-4473-3788-1 ePdf

Cover design by Hayes Design
Front cover image: Ethiopian children © scx
Printed and bound in Great Britain by CPI Group (UK) Ltd, Croydon, CR0 4YY
Policy Press uses environmentally responsible print partners

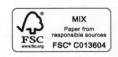

Contents

List of figures, tables, and boxes

Figures

Tables

Boxes

Preface

Few issues in the world cry out for attention as much as the tragic condition of health care in so much of Africa. From a recent and authoritative report issued by the Center for Strategic and International Studies (CSIS) in Washington DC, titled *Public Health in Africa*, it is estimated that Africa carries 24% of the world's diseases even though it only comprises 13% of the world's population (Cooke 2009).

Given the links that exist between society and health care, and the importance of religion and world view to society, the study of these things together is likely to enhance understanding of them. In fact, we take as our starting point the concept of the Social Determinants of Health—factors emphasized by the World Health Organization on its website. According to the World Health Organization (2017), "the determinants of health include: the social and economic environment; the physical environment, and the person's individual characteristics and behaviours." Our analysis takes into account the physical environments in which Africans across the continent live, the religious beliefs (where relevant) of these citizens, and each state's level of poverty, yielding a fuller account of the citizens' health status than any one factor alone. Among the factors referred to in the Social Determinants of Health on the World Health Organization website is that of culture, in which "beliefs of the family and community all affect health." Clearly, religious beliefs are an important part of that measure. Another helpful point about the Social Determinants of Health framework is that "blaming individuals for having poor health or crediting them for having good health is clearly inappropriate" (World Health Organization 2017). In other words, the social and economic environments of these three African countries classified as "low income," the physical environment, and individual predispositions all interact with each other. We are interested in identifying at what point in the chain of interactions, if at all, religious beliefs affect attitudes or beliefs about, or the availability of, access to health care in Uganda, Mozambique, and Ethiopia, along with African states in general.

The CSIS report observes at its outset that religious organizations play a role in combating disease. The remainder of its pages, however, are relatively quiet about how that occurs and what might be done to promote greater access to health care. What, then, is the role played by religion regarding health care in Africa?

This book begins to answer that question by assessing how religious beliefs in the three African countries of Uganda, Mozambique, and

Ethiopia affect health care. Given the complex nature of this project, a three-way collaboration is in place. Each member of the team is an expert in one or even two of the following essential areas: African society and politics, health care, and religion. For example, Robert Lloyd has visited many African states for research purposes and even lived in Mozambique—he is fluent in the version of Portuguese spoken there—as a former employee of a faith-based non-governmental organization (NGO). Melissa Haussman is a comparativist in Political Science who has published on the topics of federalism, multi-level governance, and women's reproductive rights and policies. Patrick James has traveled to a number of African countries and also served as director of a research project on religion and global governance.

This book is intended for those with interests in Africa, health care, and religion. The volume should also appeal to scholars in any social science and interdisciplinary fields, such as gender studies, because of the nature of the work. Given its focus on health care, the research in this book resides at the intersection of the natural and social sciences, which means that the audience could be broader still. For example, scholars with interests in science-related policy areas might want to read the book as well. We also hope to convey our results, as noted earlier, to those in various policy communities.

Obtaining data in Africa, as a general rule, is logistically difficult and relatively expensive. Making this task even more difficult is the topic we chose. This book, with its interdisciplinary focus on health, religion, politics, and money—all the private and contentious topics that we had been taught as children not to publicly discuss with others—boldly charts a course through undiscovered territory. No single book in print, to the best of our knowledge, combines an interest in religion, health care, and Africa. (Articles and book chapters, however, do exist.) The process of research for this study explains why such books appear to be absent: the high difficulty level in terms of accessing sources on the ground, along with the required expertise, which is substantial and diverse. These challenges have probably discouraged such projects in the past. However, with excellent connections on the ground in Ethiopia and Uganda through the Institute for Global Health (IGH) at the University of Southern California (USC) and a participant with many years of experience from living in Mozambique, our team managed to obtain extraordinary access to information that facilitates an in-depth, book-length exposition. Our interviews in Uganda, Mozambique, and Ethiopia included government officials, religious NGOs, and health-care providers. This work is the first of its kind: an investigation of religion and health care in Africa that is informed by the most relevant examination of the existing literature and on-the-ground interviews with individuals and organizations most familiar with the issues.

Under the leadership of Dr Jonathan Samet, Director of the IGH, and Dr Patrick James, Director of the Center of International Studies (2006–2015), the University of Southern California initiated this project—which has now borne fruit in this present volume—to learn more about the link between health services and religion. One of the underlying reasons for this proposed research agenda is the impact of religious beliefs on polio eradication programs in sub-Saharan Africa (particularly Nigeria, where opposition to polio vaccinations in 2003 by governors and religious leaders led to renewed outbreaks of the disease). A second reason is the completion of previous research on the relationship of religion with international relations (see, among others, Johnston and Sampson 1995). In many ways, this work extends that earlier project, which established that religious belief, politics, and health care are interrelated issues of great salience.

We are grateful to Cody Brown for outstanding research assistance. He carried out challenging tasks above and beyond the call of duty. Cody is a fine scholar in his own right and many pages of this volume are much better than they would otherwise have been because of his superb work. We note in particular his ability to locate studies on topics out of the research mainstream, along with excellent judgment about the utilization of empirical source material.

Indira Persad from the Center for International Studies provided valuable help as well in terms of travel arrangements and work on the manuscript. Therese Anders, Kalanzi Rukia, Marina Tolchinsky, Somto Ugwueze, and referees from Bristol University Press gave insightful critiques, and Nicolas De Zamoraczy drew attention to valuable references.

One very special event, which helped this book in so many ways, took place at the conference of the International Studies Association (ISA) in Quito, Ecuador. A roundtable held at that ISA conference, in July 2018, produced invaluable commentaries from both the audience and other participants. We are grateful to Amy Adamczyk, Dauda Aubabar, Emmanuel Balogun, Jane Parpart, and Tim Shaw for insightful responses to the draft manuscript. Odilile Ayodele, who attended the roundtable, also provided thoughtful reactions.

Most notably through a sabbatical year for Patrick James, the School of International Relations at USC (University of Southern California) supported this project in ways too numerous to mention. Pepperdine University assisted this project through the granting of both time and finances to Robert Lloyd. Finally, we appreciate our editor, Laura Vickers-Rendall, and her team at Policy Press of Bristol University Press very much indeed. This book is so much better because of the help we have received along the way—the problems that remain are our responsibility alone.

1

Religion, health care, and Africa

Overview

Few studies focus on the influence of religion or a religious world view with regard to health care in Africa. An impressive policy review on health care in Africa by Cooke (2009), for example, acknowledges the importance of religion but does not go beyond that point in exploring the connection. A recent and valuable study of health-care policy in Africa acknowledged the importance of spirituality, but its agenda on state and society only touched upon religious institutions (Gros 2016: 179). The intersection point of religion, health care, and Africa emerges as a principal item for the research agenda on well-being.

Among other aspects of this book, the primary argument is that religious beliefs (including, by extension, the beliefs of those who do not necessarily profess religious beliefs) are central to an integrated world view. This world view shapes Africans' understanding of the world and how best to respond to its complexity. Health care is an essential aspect of an individual's physical, emotional, and psychological well-being. The study examines the relationship of the physical and spiritual domains by examining how religious belief affects the provision and consumption of public health.

States sometimes cannot fulfill their social contract to citizens. Thus, dysfunctional states create an opening for religion to impact significantly on both the provision and consumption of health care in Africa. Government corruption and incompetence vary throughout the continent, but it is fair to say that no regime in Africa is free from the side effects, which include seeking public services from the private sector. This is one underlying explanation for why traditional healers, along with Faith-Inspired Institutions that provide modern medicine, turn out to be so important in the pages of this book. The other foundational reason is the importance to Africans, in seeking health care and other services, of meeting needs in a way that is in line with their religious faith. Many Africans pursue health in a holistic way— spiritual and physical needs are regarded as connected to each other.

Among Africans, the role of religion is significant across the board. The impact of religion on politics and policy in Africa is well established (Meier and Steinforth 2014). Faith-based medicine is long-standing. Some time ago, Mbiti (1969: 166, 170–171) identified traditional medicine with herbalism and, although allowing for exceptions, cast it in a generally positive light. Traditional medicine "refers to health practices, approaches, knowledge and beliefs incorporating plant, animal and mineral-based medicines, spiritual therapies, manual techniques and exercises, applied singularly or in a combination to treat, diagnose and prevent illnesses or maintain well-being" (Birhan et al 2011: 2). "In African villages," Mbiti (1969: 169) observed, "disease and misfortune are religious experiences" and it "requires a religious approach to deal with them." Yet, even otherwise comprehensive studies of health care in Africa tend to leave faith healing out of the research agenda (Gros 2016: 258).

Knowledge about African-based humanitarian organizations, another important part of the story regarding religion and health, is also limited. This is true despite a sustained history of involvement from missionary hospitals (Olivier and Wodon 2012c: 1; Gros 2016: 154). These entities, with Dr Albert Schweitzer as the most well-remembered figure among those active long ago, played an essential role in African health care from the turn of the 20th century onward (Gros 2016: 9). The history of Christian evangelism to Africa, and, by extension, spiritual and physical healing, extends back to the early Church. The New Testament Book of Acts of the Apostles (Chapter 8, verses 26–39) records how Philip, an early Christian leader, met a high-level Ethiopian government official visiting Jerusalem to worship God. Through this encounter and their subsequent discussion of Jesus and the Old Testament Book of Isaiah, the Ethiopian becomes a Christian. He is baptized and subsequently returns home. Ethiopia and much of North Africa had become Christian within a few centuries of the birth of the Church at Pentecost. By the early 15th century, Portuguese Catholic missions had become established along a few coastal areas of sub-Saharan Africa.

In particular, the degree of influence of Faith-Based Organizations (also known as Faith-Inspired Institutions in the literature) on Africa in general is far from fully understood (Tolchinsky 2013).[1] According to Schmid et al (2008: 10 emphasis added; see also Budge-Reid et al 2012: 104), there is "*little data* on the faith-based contribution to health

---

[1]   Faith-Based Organizations and Faith-Inspired Institutions are subsets within the larger and familiar category of non-governmental organizations (NGOs).

and to date no comprehensive database of religious health facilities for SSA [sub-Saharan Africa] exists nor of their funders and good practice exemplars; even less is known about non-facility-based services." Recent works from the World Bank (Olivier and Wodon 2012g, 2012h, 2012i) focus on the role of faith-inspired health-care providers in Africa along multiple dimensions: (1) public–private partnerships; (2) in comparison with other sources; and (3) with respect to mapping, cost, and reach. Results from these studies, to be reviewed in detail at a later point, encourage further research on religion and health care in Africa from both academic and policy standpoints.

Health care, moreover, is rising on the agenda of the public in Africa as well. This is a natural by-product of economic stagnation and even decline for the continent; Africans can see, quite easily, the seriousness of ongoing health challenges in a setting of limited and, in some instances, even diminishing resources. According to a recent Pew Research Center survey carried out in nine African states (Wike and Simmons 2015: 2), Africans put health care, followed by education, as the highest development priority. The survey of over 9,000 respondents in nine states from March through May 2015 also happens to include two of the three states featured in the present study: Ethiopia and Uganda. In Uganda and Ethiopia, respectively, 44% and 38% of respondents identify health care as the top priority for their country—the highest of any issue. This is to be expected because, as forthcoming pages will reveal, health care is both essential and challenging to obtain.

Some limitations should be noted before the study moves along much further. The most obvious is that a sample of three states from a population of over 50 quite properly induces a sense of caution about generalizing on the basis of results from research. The three states are also located in East Africa and contain Christian majorities and a Muslim minority. With regard to interviews conducted, ethical considerations limit the sample to those with roles in the health-care sector. Providers are represented more than patients, though, of course, every person is also a seeker of health care.

For the present volume, two interrelated research questions set the agenda. The first query is: how does religion contribute to the *social* determinants of health care in each country?[2] The social determinants

---

[2]   The potential agenda regarding the overall determinants of health is vast and beyond the scope of this study. For purposes of illustration, consider the contents of one comprehensive model of the determinants of health: age, sex, and constitutional factors; individual lifestyle factors; and social and community networks/general

of health (SDOH) are defined as the "circumstances in which people grow, live, work and age, and the systems put in place to deal with illness" (World Health Organization, 2014: 88). Three dimensions are considered: (1) the nature of the providers—religious (eg Muslim, Christian, and also separated out by denomination and whether evangelical, along with traditional) or secular (ie national or local government), along with the location of provision; (2) health-seeking behaviors by various populations; and (3) the influence of religion on the public. These dimensions combine to cover the *process* through which religion is connected to health care. The other basic research question focuses on how religion is linked with desired *outcomes*: how does religion impact the countries as to moving forward (through providers, institutions, and public beliefs/behaviors) on the Millennium Development Goals (MDGs)[3] of the United Nations (UN)? Similarly, what will the effects be, post-2015, as the MDGs are subsumed into the Sustainable Development Goals (SDGs)? All African governments made a public commitment to the two preceding sets of objectives, so these are the most relevant indicators to consider in terms of health outcomes.

The eight MDGs are obviously interconnected; it is easy to imagine how pursuit of one goal might impact upon another. Several of the goals focus on health in an explicit way: Goal 4—reduce child mortality; Goal 5a—reduce maternal mortality; Goal 5b—increase access to contraception and comprehensive reproductive services; and Goal 6—combat HIV/AIDS, malaria, and other diseases.

Some of the binary connections that feed into the preceding goals are quite easy to see as well. Potentially most important for this study, in that sense, is Goal 3: promote gender equity and empower women. This goal, for instance, obviously possesses important implications, to the degree of its fulfillment, for Goals 4 and 5 in particular. An improved position for women in society, by intuition even prior to systematic research, must help along any number of dimensions impacting upon families, such as reducing child mortality. As will become apparent from subsequent chapters, all of that is influenced by religious world view.

Another important connection with the explicitly health-oriented objectives concerns Goal 1, which seeks to eradicate extreme poverty

---

socio-economic, cultural, and environmental conditions (agriculture and food production, education, work environment, living and working conditions, unemployment, water and sanitation, health-care services, and housing) (Mikkonen and Raphael 2010: 9; see also Raphael 2009: 5).

[3]   http://mdgs.un.org/unsd/mdg/Data.aspx

and hunger. Health is impacted in so many ways by poverty—the inability to prevent the spread of disease and losses through infant mortality due to the lack of care come immediately to mind, along with other unfortunate connections. Still further connections emerge with Goal 2, which pursues universal primary education. Knowledge constitutes power in the domain of health, notably, in relation to practices that can head off illness. Furthermore, it is easy to see how Goal 7—ensuring environmental sustainability—is relevant to health as well. Air pollution, for instance, is a menace to good health.

Finally, Goal 8—develop a global partnership for development—is panoramic and intersects with all of the other goals. It stands as an overarching objective, the achievement of which is certain to help with the MDGs that are specific to health.[4]

One feature of this volume, intellectually speaking, will be a special focus on women's health. MDGs 2 and 4–6 are addressed in detail by the three country chapters in order to assess changes in women's health care since 2000. Attention is paid to: the interaction of the MDG goals and targets for sub-Saharan Africa (including the three countries emphasized in this volume); the role of religion in beliefs and the provision of health care; and outcomes for African citizens, disaggregated by gender, in our three case studies. Thus, as the World Health Organization recommends, both system- and individual-level factors are investigated.

UN member states approved the Millennium Declaration in 2000. This multilateral effort aimed at improving the economic and social well-being of the world's poorer countries by 2015. Five of the Declaration's eight goals related in whole or in part to health. The next year, the heads of member states of the African Union, while meeting in the Nigerian capital of Abuja, subsequently reached an agreement on increasing health spending. The Abuja Declaration on HIV/AIDS, Tuberculosis and Other Related Infectious Diseases, among a number of items, stated that national health budgets would increase to a targeted amount of 15% of the total government budget. The African leaders also called for wealthier donor countries to increase their foreign assistance to 0.7% of their gross national income. Taken together, these

---

[4]   The more recently articulated SDGs remain at a very early stage of implementation. For such reasons, the emphasis in this study is on the MDGs, which have been in place since 2000. An introduction to the SDGs, which involved a more "collaborative process," appears in Krishnamani (2015a). For valuable overviews regarding the MDGs and the three states covered in the present study, see MDG Global Database (2015a, 2015b, 2015c).

two measures would increase the funding available for health spending in African countries. The African leaders also called for forgiveness on debt owed to donor states and multilateral organizations, a major issue at that time, so African states could redirect funds to the social sector. By 2015, the Abuja Declaration had not reached the intended targets for health spending. Nonetheless, some measures, such as the President's Emergency Plan for AIDS Relief (PEPFAR)—authorized by the US Congress as the U.S. Leadership Against HIV/AIDS, Tuberculosis, and Malaria Act 2003—represented a major increase in donor funding for HIV/AIDS prevention and treatment (Organization of African Unity 2001; World Health Organization 2011).

In related fashion, the Assembly of the African Union in Maputo, Mozambique, adopted the Maputo Protocol to the African Charter on Human and Peoples' Rights on the Rights of Women in Africa in 2003. The Protocol took effect in November 2005 after 15 countries had signed on. So far, 49 of the African Union countries have signed the Protocol, while 37 of them have ratified and deposited it, becoming "States' Parties" to the Protocol. Developed in meetings held in Africa the same year as the Beijing Conference on Women's Rights, the Protocol requires states to take measures to end female genital mutilation (FGM) and ensure women's autonomy in contraceptive use and reproductive decisions in general. A list of articles from the Protocol includes:

> the elimination of discrimination against women; the right to dignity; the right to life, integrity and security of the person; the right to access to justice and equal protection before the law; the right to participation in political and decision-making processes; the right to peace; and the right to protection in armed conflicts. (Sigsworth and Kumalo 2016: 2)

Many of the Protocol's guarantees are consistent with the Convention on the Elimination of all Forms of Discrimination Against Women, the Beijing Platform, and the gender-focused MDGs 2–6. Among the chapter-length cases included in this study, Mozambique and Uganda signed and ratified, while Ethiopia signed, the Protocol. Based on two separate information sources, of the 55 states in the African Union, 37 have ratified the Protocol, with 49 members merely signing it (FIDH 2013; African Union 2010).

Over and beyond the MDGs (now SDGs) and Maputo Protocol, it is possible to point to the declaration of the "African Women's Decade" of 2010–2020 on November 8, 2010. The launch included African heads of state and government, African Union ministers, representatives of the UN, civil society, development groups, and the private sector, among others (UN NGLS 2010). As with the MDGs and Maputo Protocol, the African Women's Decade brings global attention to the many areas of civil, social, economic, and political rights needing more work to achieve gender equality. The 10 areas of focus for the African Women's Decade have included:

> Fighting Poverty and Promoting Economic Empowerment of Women and Entrepreneurship; Agriculture and Food Security; Health, Maternal Mortality and HIV/AIDS; Education, Science and Technology; Environment and Climate Change; Peace and Security and Violence against Women; Governance and Legal Protection; Finance and Gender Budgets; Women in Decision-Making Positions; and Young Women's Movement. (UN NGLS 2010)

Clearly, the three multi-level instruments mentioned earlier, with central foci on many aspects of gender equality, draw on prior work such as the UN Declaration of Human Rights, the Convention on the Elimination of all Forms of Discrimination Against Women, the Cairo Programme of Action on Population and Development, and the Beijing Platform on Women. Women involved in global rights-seeking organizations have been active on multiple fronts, so it is possible to see various frameworks in operation at the same time (for example Maputo, the MDGs, and the African Women's Decade). The multiplicity of frameworks speaks to strategic decisions by women's movement activists, plus those affiliated with the UN and African Union, to keep issues related to gender equality alive and on the "front burner" of international policymaking.

Since the early 21st century, the World Economic Forum has constructed a global "gender gap" based on parity between women and men (1.0) or lack of parity (0) from four sets of factors: political participation; health and survival; educational attainment; and economic participation and opportunity (World Economic Forum 2016). Out of the 144 countries included on the composite global index, Mozambique ranked 21st in 2016 with a score of 0.750 (out of a possible 1), Uganda placed 61st with an overall score of 0.704, and Ethiopia came in at 109th with a score of 0.662 (World Economic Forum 2016: 10–11).

7

Make Every Woman Count (2016), in their Mid-Term Review of the African Women's Decade, sees uneven implementation for some of the multi-level commitments across Africa (and East Africa, for present purposes). While the Mid-Term Review notes that maternal mortality has been dropping in the East Africa region, it also observes that, "as many East African countries have weak health-care systems, more needs to be done to ensure women's safety" (Make Every Woman Count 2016: 42). Other issues that the Mid-Term Review identified in 2016, after the "end" date of the MDGs in 2015, included that Ethiopia routinely violates provisions in the Convention on the Elimination of all Forms of Discrimination Against Women despite having ratified it. While Ethiopia included FGM in its Criminal Code in 2005, there is no stand-alone provision against it and rates remain high. Specifically regarding MDG 5a, as of 2016, Ethiopia reported only 10% of births being attended by skilled personnel. Finally, regarding MDGs 2 and 3, Uganda and Ethiopia still had high rates of teenage marriage, with 40% of women in Uganda and 27% in Ethiopia having been married by age 18 (Make Every Woman Count 2016: 41–42).

Gender is critical as an intervening variable related to prior health, health-seeking behavior, and the future of health outcomes for individuals and groups in the following ways. The changing stances over time of the governments in the three countries that we have studied , and inconsistent access to health interventions in a timely manner (particularly during pregnancy and childbirth), affect women in ways in which men are not affected.

As with religion, the interaction of gender at an individual and collective level with health practices, including those of health-providing institutions, is not linear and the same within one country, at different time periods, or across the three countries that we discuss. The SDOH framework is used to introduce a concept of *social disadvantage*, whereby individual and collective scores on various health indices (such as obesity, tobacco and drug use, toxins such as asbestos or coal fires inhaled in living spaces, lack of self-control over women's fertility, etc) are all known to affect women and men, the elderly and children, and rural and urban inhabitants differently. When individuals present themselves to a health practitioner (whether religious or secular) and/ or institution, their experience will be preconditioned by their life experiences, and the ability to access better health in the future rests on their experiences to date.

The reason for integrating the MDGs with SDOH in our conceptual model is that on the MDG indicators, women were shown to have lifelong deficiencies in many African countries relating to empowerment experiences, namely, access to education and their decision-making status in their relationships. As is discussed in the chapters, access to education is one of the key determinants in showing whether women will feel confident in accessing health care, particularly sexual and reproductive health, on their own. It is also crucial in allowing girls to reject FGM and child marriage. FGM and child marriage, along with the lack of consistent visits to SRH (Sexual and Reproductive Health) practitioners during their lives, are some of the key reasons for maternal deaths and fistulas, as cited in the MDG, African Union, United Nations Children's Fund (UNICEF), United Nations Development Programme (UNDP), and Guttmacher studies (among others) cited in this book. The endemic problems of child marriage, FGM, HIV infection, and lack of timely access to health care by (often) rural-dwelling individuals has been reinforced by wars and emigration to refugee camps in the countries under study. Finally, at times, traditional practices regarding marriage, which interrelate with traditional African religion, especially in rural areas, have encouraged early marriage through the practice of lobolo or bride price. Early marriage, when it is not combined with regular access to comprehensive reproductive health care, does not bode well for the mother's physical or mental health.

Not surprisingly, there have also been critiques of the multi-level instruments. With respect to the MDGs, one criticism relates to overly ambitious goals set in place for the world's poorest and least-resourced countries (Clemens and Moss 2005). Take the first goal—halving poverty by 2015—as an example. Clemens and Moss (2005) point out that for Africa to have done that between 2000 and 2015, the countries would have required an annual economic growth rate higher than 7%. Only seven of the 153 countries for which they had data managed that between 1990 and 2005 (Clemens and Moss 2005: 2). Another critique, accompanying action by the global women's health movement, pertains to the lack of a reproductive care emphasis in MDG 5, which originally focused on increasing the percentage of live births and healthy children. Added in 2005, MDG 5b called for "universal access to reproductive health care" around the world by 2015.

Church organizations have likewise criticized the multi-level frameworks crafted by regional and international conferences on population and gender equality. Speaking out most often as a critic is the Catholic Church (Haussman 2005). The Vatican is a member of the UN and possesses access to intervene, for example, in the platform-writing process. One strategy that the Vatican consistently uses is to "bracket" language with which it disagrees. Future conferences are forced to take up that terminology before attending to other business. Similarly, in 2007, Pope Benedict criticized the Maputo Protocol for its focus on gender equality, in consistent fashion with Vatican action at the UN since the 1980s and the Nairobi Conference in particular (Hambuba 2013).

Africa is home to many of the states from around the world that are classified as fragile or failed—an observation in line with the preceding discussion of limited achievements vis-a-vis MDGs. This designation means that inhabitants "live more or less beyond the meaningful reach of a central government" (Menkhaus 2014: 142–143). More specifically, state failure is "the inability of a state to perform the essential functions of statehood: tax, protect its territory, maintain internal order, define and enforce property rights, provide social services, and conduct diplomacy" (Gros 2016: 7). This problem is particularly acute in Africa. Some of the worst civil wars in history have occurred on the continent within living memory; the Congo is one such instance (Kisangani 2012). Quinn (2016: 306) assesses the institutions of sub-Saharan Africa in particular as "relatively weak." The numbers here are unequivocal: the World Bank Index of government effectiveness for 2014 (along a scale from −2.5 to +2.5) reveals world and sub-Saharan averages of 0 and −0.815, respectively (Quinn 2016: 307). The three states in the present study all appear in relatively high categories along the Fragile States Index for 2014. Among the eight categories, none is at the highest two of "very high alert" and "high alert." However, Ethiopia and Uganda appear in the third category, "alert," and Mozambique is in the fourth category of "very high warning" (Quinn 2016: 308). In other words, out of seven categories, all three of the countries included in this study appear in the top half of the eight-category scale regarding fragile states.

Research is accumulating on the unfortunate implications of political instability and inadequate health care in tandem with each other. One causal linkage is from involvement in armed conflict to a range of detrimental health-related effects, such as the destruction of infrastructure and the creation of refugees (Iqbal 2010). Cause and effect can also be bidirectional: insecurity about survival can encourage a government to provide more public services in order to enhance stability. Greater stability, in turn, will enhance the ability to offer services (Anders 2016).

Given limitations on government performance and the important consequences of the failure to provide public services, it becomes appropriate for this study to include both state and society in its investigation of health care. Governments in troubled states will not be the whole story when it comes to health-care provision. Instead, problematic states—and many in Africa meet this description—rely on groups in society to pick up after them in essential sectors. With regard to health care, it is certain that much can be learned through consultation with religious entities given their tradition of concern for the well-being of the poorest members of society. As will become apparent, religion is perhaps the single most important and under-studied aspect of society in Africa when it comes to telling the story of how needs unmet by government are addressed in ways that lie at least partially and even sometimes fully beyond its grasp. *The bottom line of this study is that religion impacts significantly on health in Africa.* This impact can be through religion's impact on personal behavior and societal norms and taboos, as well as institutionalized religion's role in health-care provision. Traditional healers are also part of this mix. So, too, are foreign non-governmental organizations (NGOs), bilateral aid, domestic NGOs, local churches, and churches helping hospitals with international support.

This study is the first of its kind at book length, so it will be neither surprising nor disappointing if more questions are raised than answered along the way. In a concrete sense, developing rather than testing ideas is more appropriate for a study with in-depth information on three cases out of more than 50 in Africa, the geographic domain of immediate interest.

With an unapologetically inductive approach, this study works toward a conceptual model of health care. Presented in Chapter 6, the model is a point of culmination of the case studies in Chapters 3–5. The conceptual model begins with the concept of supply and demand. Production and consumption of health care are linked in the model. Government, civil society, and citizens are all essential in how that plays out. The model incorporates: (1) international-level support; and (2) state (and modern and traditional) services. Health-seeking behavior takes place within the context of availability just described. The preceding aspects of the conceptual model are identified, in turn, through the application of findings from the chapters that focus on Uganda, Mozambique, and Ethiopia. The "bottom line" of the model is that religion is pervasive in how health care is provided and consumed in the three African states included in the initial sample.

This chapter proceeds in three additional sections. The next section conveys concept formation. Africa, religion, and health are covered in turn. The section that follows focuses on the intellectual context of the study. Relevant interdisciplinary fields—Religious Studies, African Studies, and Health Studies—are introduced. The present investigation is situated at the intersection of these concepts and fields. The final section outlines the subsequent chapters of this volume.

Concept Formation: Africa, Religion, and Health

In terms of physical geography, Africa comprises the world's second-largest continent, bounded by the Mediterranean Sea on its north, the Indian Ocean to the East, and the Atlantic Ocean on its western reaches. Africa's land mass is not uniform, but varies from tropical rainforest, through savannah, to desert. Vast plains exist along with mountain ranges. In both the farthest north and south, the climate is Mediterranean. The huge Sahara Desert, into which the US could easily fit, marks the traditional divide between North Africa and sub-Saharan Africa. Yet, the Sahara itself may be imagined as a basin: one vast sea of sand that links north and south along its more fertile shores. Another way to describe the area is as the location for the Sahel, or Sahelian states, and it is important not to oversimplify the preceding point of division because of the sheer range of countries touched by the desert.

Human geography on the continent is equally diverse, adding even more complexity to understanding the concept of Africa. Some one billion people live in Africa, mostly as farmers in its fertile valleys. Large mega-cities, such as Cairo, Lagos, and Kinshasa, however, are increasingly becoming a major feature of life for Africans. Northern Africa is predominantly Arab and Mediterranean in culture, but it retains the influence of Berbers in the Maghreb region of North-West Africa. Egypt's lifeblood, the Nile River, originates in the eastern part of Ethiopia (Blue Nile) and far to the south from Lake Albert, which borders the Democratic Republic of Congo and Uganda (White Nile). The Nile is a part of Africa, which wholly depends on it for life, but Egyptians are often associated more with the Middle East than Africa. Ethiopians and Somalians are similarly quite closely culturally related to the Arabian Peninsula. In sub-Saharan Africa—sometimes called tropical Africa or Black Africa—colonialism produced successor states where French, English, and Portuguese culture and language retain their influence.

Finally, the concept of Africa is not static, but dynamic. In just half a century, most of Africa has gone from being a part of the European colonial system to becoming fragmented into a large number of independent states. Some states, such as Botswana, Mauritius, and Tunisia, have thrived during all or much of independence. Others, like the Democratic Republic of Congo and Somalia, have failed (partially or fully) as states. For two generations after independence in the early 1960s, Africa remained economically stagnant. In the past decade, by contrast, many African states have been among the fastest growing in the world. Africa is both modern and traditional, international and local.

Within this geographical context, religion, another one of the book's central concepts, makes its home. Africa is a complex concept even in matters of faith. Northern Africa is predominantly Muslim and Africa south of the Sahel (the southern area bordering the Sahara Desert) is primarily a mix of Christian, Muslim, and traditional religions. Yet, for centuries, Northern Africa had also been home to vibrant Christian communities and leaders. In sub-Saharan Africa, the Swahili Coast running along the Indian Ocean from Somalia to Northern Mozambique developed into a fusion of Arab, Muslim, and Black African cultures. Both Islam and Christianity have evangelized a continent already deeply religious. Animism and traditional healing, in various locations, also factor significantly into the profile of religion intersecting with health. These beliefs have been remembered and, as will be seen later in the book, retain a major impact on the African continent, its people, and their attitudes and behavior.

Any search for a definition of religion will face great difficulty—a point that seems obvious by intuition but is also endorsed by experts in the field (Byrne 1988: 5).[5] "Religion," as introduced by Turner (1981: 1), "is a human activity and experience that is liable to be interwoven with all aspects of human life, and its study therefore requires, sooner or later, all the human sciences." The need to look at religion from many different directions is embedded within formal definitions. Take, for instance, the effort from Byrne (1988: 7):

> a religion is an institution with a complex of theoretical, practical, sociological and experiential dimensions, which is distinguished by characteristic objects (gods or sacred things), goals (salvation or ultimate good) and functions (giving an overall meaning to life or providing the identity or cohesion of a social group).

---

[5]   Some even dismiss efforts toward formal definition, with one argument being that religions exist, rather than religion per se. Self-identification of religious groupings through thought or action becomes the effective point of definition (Hinnells 2010: 6).

Religions are belief systems that include a complex mixture of myth and symbol, along with laws and values (Kaufman 2017). Religion is, in a word, multifaceted.

Consider the views of Moyser (2010: 456; see also Malley 2013: 219) on the importance of religion for the domain of public policy in particular:

> Contrary to the expectations of those who thought religion would fade from political life, this has not happened in the modern era. Religion continues as a source of authority and guidance for political action around the globe, while political leaders, for their part, have to devise strategies that take those religious claims into account.

The preceding allusions to the end of faith refer to observations from epic theorists, such as Marx and Weber, who saw religion as destined to disappear as science advanced and provided explanations for the unknown. When recalling expert forecasts from the 1960s onward that religion would decline, Hinnells (2010: 10) offers a pithy summation: "We were wrong!" (see also Hatzpoulos and Petito 2003: 1; Haynes 2013: 29). He then confirmed the ongoing "massive power" of religion (Hinnells 2010: 6; see also Moyser 2010: 445). Observations today about the significance of religion in general and for politics and policy in particular are legion. Religion possesses "cultural power," with an "immense and sustained impact" on the identity, values, and understandings at the community level; moreover, its ideas, symbols, institutions, and personnel affect politics and governance significantly (Moyser 2010: 457, 445; see also Fox and Sandler 2004). Religion, in sum, plays an essential role in public policy—especially through the sanction of the "should" or the "ought." It informs moral codes as well as the laws of society.

Religion may be of importance to believers today, but what are its prospects for the future? Might it still be on the way out, as Marx and Weber anticipated long ago? The basic answer is "no." This assessment is borne out by a wide range of evidence assembled from the World Values Survey and reported comprehensively by Norris and Inglehart (2004). Religion is holding its own or on the rise in most of the world, geographically and demographically speaking, with exceptions in Western Europe and a few other locations. A basic explanation for the resurgence of religion is that it is a form of response to effects from globalization; millions of people look to faith for reassurance in a world of rapid and even threatening change. This causal mechanism is borne out by the pattern of religious revival; religions showing the highest levels of increase are relatively directive in their beliefs, with Pentecostalism and variants of Islam leading the way. Strong religion, put simply, is on the rise (Almond et al 2003). This is especially true in the developing world, where secular modernity as an ideology among many governments is regarded by the public as a failure in terms of economic performance and justice (Fox 2013: 23). Moreover, traditional and alternative healing has been on the rise around the globe over the last decade (Birhan et al 2011: 2).

This review of religion as a concept concludes without a formal definition. Given the interview-based method within the case studies, relying on self-designation rather than imposing a template makes the most sense. In other words, the goal is to study religion in an inclusive way that facilitates the most insight, as opposed to an investigation that seeks to advance concept formation in and of itself. African religions, it should be noted, are interwoven with world view—the rule rather than the exception. For example, most diseases are seen in Africa as being created by malevolent spirits or thoughts (Mbiti 1969).[6]

Health as a testable measure, according to Raphael (2009), is not a traditional, binary variable that an individual either possesses or not. In the SDOH paradigm, the state of health is an intervening variable, influenced by an individual's socio-economic status and ability to access health care. Extremely important to note is that the structure of the health-care system is a fundamental component of the SDOH framework (Raphael 2009: xvii): "pioneering Canadian (but also other countries') public health units have worked to shift the discussion away from biomedical and behavioural health risks toward emphasizing living conditions as the primary determinants of individual and population health." Subsequent chapters confirm that action or inaction on the MDGs is implicated directly in whether citizens of the states concerned can access necessary health care and thus score reasonably well on such indicators.

Health, like religion, is an ambiguous, changing concept in itself. The World Health Organization defined health in the Preamble to its 1948 founding Constitution as a "complete state of physical, mental and social well-being, not just the absence of infirmity." While this definition has been lauded for moving away from a negative definition of health, some believe that it is time to reframe the concept (Huber et al 2011). Huber et al (2011: 1) assert that the World Health

---

6   As an interesting side point, this feature may make at least some conversions to US-style fundamentalist religions more appealing in the region.

Organization definition requires "total health, all the time." While the most prevalent diseases in the mid-20th century were acute ones that had to be medically managed in an acute care setting, Huber et al (2011: 1) point to the fact that populations in both the Global North and South live with chronic, long-term diseases. In this frame of reference, "chronic diseases account for most of the expenditures of the healthcare system, putting pressure on its sustainability" (Huber et al 2011: 1). Huber et al (2011) also fault the requirement for reaching a "complete" state of health, arguing that this is impossible.

Huber et al (2011: 2) observe that operational definitions of health are needed for "measurement purposes, research, and evaluating interventions." They propose "constructing health frames that systematize different operational needs," such as differentiating between the health statuses of individuals and general populations. Measurements "should relate to health as the ability to adapt and to self-manage" (Huber et al 2011: 2). In that regard, the World Health Organization has developed ways to measure gradations of health (rather than an absolute presence or absence) and these tools should be used more (Huber et al 2011).

Huber et al's (2011) call for ways to measure "quality of life and sense of wellbeing" is quite relevant to the research project undertaken in this book. An individual's quality of life and ability to access resources (including health care) are often intertwined with their degree of education and income, as per the SDOH model. Quality of life is also measured in terms of how well the three African countries under study have done in reaching MDGs 2 and 4–6 regarding gender differences in education and health.

Furthermore, the desire to measure quality of life and sense of well-being relates back to an early framework developed by psychologists in the 1950s: the "health beliefs" model. In part, that model, used by the US Public Health Service, incorporated the idea that individuals will respond to their illnesses based on how the concept of health is perceived by them and their reference groups. Social-psychological expositions, such as Almond and Verba's (1965) *The Civic Culture*, explained people's willingness to vote based on their sense of efficacy vis-a-vis the political system; similarly, the "health beliefs" model uses individual and group efficacy to account for why people do not access health-care resources when they need them (Becker 1974). The SDOH framework of the World Health Organization and the "health beliefs" model will combine effectively in the three case-study chapters to show how the health-care system itself, depending on its location and funding, can serve as either a barrier or conduit to accessibility.

State-of-the-art thinking, which emphasizes a comprehensive approach toward well-being, is foreshadowed by the United Nations Development Programme (1994) identification of seven domains: economic, health, food, environmental, personal, community, and political. The Centre for Health Sciences Training, Research and Development (2013: 6; see also Takemi et al 2008a, 2008b) links health to the overarching concept of human security, notably, in the context of Africa.[7] In recent years, the capabilities approach, a natural descendant of the preceding perspective on human development and certainly not at odds with human security, is gaining traction. Hodgett and Clark (2011) point out that the capabilities approach includes a multidimensional sense of well-being; in tandem, the idea of a good life can vary from one society to the next. This new trend in research provides further support to the direction of the present study, which adopts the SDOH as its overall point of view. Health care should be studied in a way that emphasizes its place within the totality of human existence.

One further definition, namely, health care, is essential before moving to the next set of concepts. In a compelling study of Africa, Gros (2016: 2) provides the following definition: health care "refers to the science, art, skills, beliefs, and practices that are brought to bear on the disease prevention, cure, and the promotion of good mental and physical health, the efficacy of which is not always readily apparent." This comprehensive definition is in line with the perspective adopted by the SDOH. As will become apparent from the subsequent case-study chapters on health care, the definition's emphasis on both mind and body, along with science and art, works especially well in an African context.

Intellectual context: religious studies, African studies, and health studies

One way to begin the discussion of Religious Studies is to stipulate what it is *not*. Sutherland (1988: 30–31) observes that "the study of religion(s) is not, for example, the study of what God is, but is the study of what men and women *believe* or *say* that God is." Thus, the centroid of Religious Studies is not theology, but, instead, the pursuit of answers to a set of questions that focus on knowledge, understanding, where to place attention, and what methods to apply in learning about respective

---

[7] The concept of human security is not without controversy; for an introduction to the debate, see Paris (2001).

belief systems (Sutherland 1988: 29).[8] Along similar lines, many years later, it is asserted that "the very core of the study of religion consists in *identifying and analyzing worldviews* in their various diachronic and synchronic ramifications" (Vernoff 2013: 61, emphasis added). The study of belief systems and their impact on the world might be regarded as a summing up of the consensus that exists regarding the content of Religious Studies over the long term.

Origins and functions are the focal points for Religious Studies in practice (Segal 2010: 75; see also Capps 1995; Capps 2013). These subjects demonstrate continuity from the era of the epic theorists of the late 19th and early 20th centuries, when religion, as noted earlier, tended to be dismissed as an epiphenomenal mechanism of social control. Thus, once upon a time, the potential value of religion to elites as a means of controlling the masses stood as the account of its origins and ongoing essential function. With the unexpected persistence and even resurgence of religion, however, the preceding unidimensional view no longer holds sway. Religious Studies, in all likelihood, does not need a universal category of religion to be viable as an academic field (Alles 2008: 313). Instead, religion is regarded as more multifaceted in its roles at the individual and collective levels. As a result, the essence of Religious Studies is pluralism with regard to the disciplines involved, with a range of terminology and methods as natural side effects (Turner 1981: 1; Sutherland 1988: 32, 39; Capps 1995: 331; Alles 2010: 41; Hoffman 2010: 236). Capps (1995: 331) sums up the diversity of contemporary Religious Studies:

> religious studies is a multiform subject-field within which a variety of disciplines are employed to treat a multiplicity of issues, interests, and topics. Religious studies has no single subject, nor does it sanction any one method or approach. Rather, the subject is multiple, and the methods of approach are numerous.

Religious Studies thus emerges as an interdisciplinary field, with contributions that range from anthropology, through political science, to economics and beyond.

---

[8]   Raschke (2013: 52) describes Religious Studies as the phoenix rising from the ashes of Christian theology, and Alles (2010: 39) observes that the study of religion in a non-theological sense dates back "in earnest" until only after the Second World War.

Intellectual diversity is a strength of the study of religion, with ideas and methods from many disciplines brought to bear. Coherence, however, then becomes a challenge. The basic point of contention within Religious Studies, put simply, concerns the presumed value of phenomenological approaches versus those nested within the social sciences, most notably, rational choice and cognitive models (Chitando 2005: 313; Alles 2010: 50–51; Vernoff 2013: 57). Theorists of the former persuasion see the origin and function of a belief system as distinctly religious, whereas those of the latter type view religion more in the role of an independent variable or cause leading to some effect (Segal 2010: 77, 78).

From one side of the debate, critics of the trend toward social science wonder: "where in our scheme of education and scholarship do we make place for the religious imagination?" (Neusner 2013: 41; see also Segal 2013: 86). Sharma (2013: 83) labels the social-scientific approach as "reductionistic" and offers an analogy to point out that religion is something more than just a variable within some network of cause and effect: "It is not possible to see without light, but vision is not a property of light but of the eye." This comparison effectively endorses a phenomenological approach toward the subject matter of Religious Studies, in opposition to a social-scientific focus on networks of variables and the identification of causes and effects among them.

Social-scientific critiques of Religious Studies as practiced in its initial decades mounted from the advent of the behavioral revolution onward. Criticism focused on phenomenology, which had been the standard approach, and labeled it as "religionist, idealistic and unscientific" (Chitando 2005: 310). Hoffman (2010: 236) adds that the phenomenology of religion is attacked because of an "unspecified subject of inquiry, theological slant, subjectivism, empirical groundlessness, and also methodological contradictions." The foundation of such a critique, philosophically speaking, is positivism. As in so many other fields, the basic point of contention in Religious Studies today comes down to interpretive versus empirical approaches. For that reason, disagreement persists in Religious Studies, but perhaps in a way that is beneficial overall. Scholarship is divided between cultural studies and scientific approaches (Alles 2010: 50, 51). Yet, it is not hard to argue a place for *both* and, in terms of method, the present volume reflects that belief.

Case studies in Chapters 3–5 include interviews with those active in the health sector of each state. This reflective material is conveyed against the backdrop of primary and secondary literature that encompasses quantitative and qualitative data. The research design is, in a word, multi-method. Thus, as a manifestation of Religious

Studies, the present work is based within the social sciences but with an appreciation for the essential role of interview material in a context, namely, Africa, where data collection is especially challenging.

Multidisciplinary study of a region such as Africa, to begin, is included in what is commonly called area studies. Area studies grew in number and importance following the end of the Second World War. The new position of the US as a superpower in the international system and the ensuing Cold War increased Washington's interest in, and backing for, specialists in regions such as Africa. Finally, entities such as the Carnegie Corporation and the Ford Foundation funded research in area studies.

African Studies, in this framework, comprises the multidisciplinary study of the African continent. The African Studies Association (2016) defines this as being a "holistic approach" that includes "all facets of Africa's political, economic, social, cultural, artistic, scientific, and environmental landscapes." The study of Africa, of course, preceded the Second World War, but it received new impetus during the Cold War. This stimulus coincided with, and became deepened by, Africa's decolonization and the birth of scores of independent African states in the 1950s and 1960s. Within the US, increased academic and policy interest in the continent, for example, led to the establishment of the African Studies Association in 1957.[9] The independence era in Africa led to new links between African and non-African scholars. Much of this initial research interaction, however, focused on the controversial apartheid regime of South Africa rather than the newly independent states. Research conducted by the growing body of African and Western scholars took place separately. The civil rights era of the 1960s in the US brought calls to study Africa and the African diaspora from a black perspective. Much of this energy came to be channeled into the creation of African American Studies programs at universities in the US (Martin 2011: 75).

Africa's acute economic and political crises of the 1980s and 1990s led to increased pessimism about the continent's future prospects.[10] Decreased multidisciplinary interest in African Studies also occurred during a time of increased application of ideas from the discipline of economics to Africa. This approach matched the growing push

---

[9] An excellent review of the development of African Studies appears in Martin (2011).

[10] During this period, one of the authors, for example, upon a number of occasions, was discouraged by professors from studying Africa academically as this would not provide much of a professional future.

by Western donor states for the economic reform of struggling African economies though the application of political and economic liberalization. The "Washington Consensus" is the term often used to refer to the policy prescriptions for Africa.

African Studies faces increasing challenges. These include reduced funding for multidisciplinary African Studies programs, the growing application of single-discipline economic analysis, and the perception that the academic study of Africa has become increasingly ideological. These developments have led, in part, for example, to the establishment of the Association for the Study of the Middle East and Africa as an additional scholarly and policy forum to study Africa from a broad multidisciplinary area studies perspective (ASMEA 2016).

Despite these challenges, a multidisciplinary, area-based approach such as African Studies affords a number of advantages over a single-discipline approach. Positive traits include higher awareness of local factors that affect analysis, as well as greater appreciation for the complexity of phenomena. In the three country cases examined in Chapters 3–5 of this book, it has proven critical to explain the relationship of religion with health care by examining cultural, political, economic, institutional, religious, and gender-based perspectives. Isolating any one of these elements would have led to an incomplete analysis of the topic at hand. A purely economic analysis of the provision of health in Africa, for example, would not have properly assessed the role of traditional healers or faith-based motivations in explaining human behavior. Thus, the area studies approach proves advantageous as a conceptual frame of reference for analyzing religion and health care in Africa.

Health Studies is inherently inter- and multidisciplinary. Most academic disciplines, as well as the fields of medicine, have some form of scholarly publishing related to questions of health. The "big questions" often vary, for example, in the fields of medicine. "Large-N" studies related to epidemiology and public health interventions are typical. In some social science disciplines, such as Sociology, the same is true. In the social sciences such as Political Science and History, either mixed-method or qualitative studies are often the norm.

With the rise of various social movements, Health Studies in the social sciences has taken account of justice-related issues connected to health-care provision and access. For example, Boychuk (2008) studied the development of Medicaid in the US and ended up tying its founding circumstances to racism. Olson (2010), in *The Politics of Medicaid*, examined the large gaps within which the poor fall even under that system. Comparative works in Health Studies are expanding as well (Maioni 1998; Tuohy 1999).

Many scholars of health, as with those who investigate the politics of race and poverty, look at other grounds of marginalization when discussing provision and insurance. A large literature exists on gender and health care, including authors such as Hankivsky (2012) on intersectionality and health-care provision in Canada, Haussman (2005) on the comparative politics of reproductive health-care provision in federal states, and Boyd-Judson and James (2013) on women's global health in relation to norms and state policies.

Most of the countries in the Global North (and some in the Global South) have academics who devote much of their research focus to explaining why their country, alone or in comparison, developed a given system. Most health-care systems in the 21st century are "hybrids" of what used to be seen as the mutually exclusive social, public, and private insurance systems (Tuohy 1999).

Since multi-level frameworks and actors have become ever-more important in funding and shaping the available health-care options in their member states, a whole segment of the literature has opened up, for example, on European Union (EU) directives, migration, and health-care rights. The European Social Observatory, working with the World Health Organization, publishes many series on how domestic and supranational health-care structures have evolved (or not) in keeping with current challenges (see, among others, Saltman et al 2004; Mossialos et al 2010; Sim and McKee 2011).

Just as the EU is a complex multi-level institution, so is the African Union. Unlike the well-funded European Social Observatory, holding a contract with the Open University Press, it is more difficult to get funding to research health care in Africa. A book on *Financing Health Care in Sub-Saharan Africa* appeared over two decades ago (Vogel 1993). While there are still some single- or two-country studies, it has become clear that work encompassing multiple case studies is badly needed (see Baylies and Bujra 2000; Sama and Nguyen 2008; Digby et al 2010; Boyd-Judson and James 2013). Subsequent chapters will review findings from *articles* that focus on specific aspects of religion and health care in Africa, but *books*, with rare exceptions, will not be part of that exercise.

There is ample need for a book such as ours to fill some of the gaps in knowledge about the three-way interaction of religion, health care, and Africa. This process begins with a juxtaposition of three countries not often compared to each other in the combined context of the SDOH and MDG frameworks. The study should encourage further research that is wider in scope in the quest for a compelling model of religion and health care for Africa. This agenda could expand to the developing world and matters beyond health care, with an interview-based approach at the center of research in recognition of the unique elements at work in the study of religion and policy issues.

More specifically, this book is intended to encourage further studies that focus on individual health access. The pages to come will reveal that Africans are *actors*, not just those acted upon. Pre-existing beliefs about the role played by providers of traditional health—perhaps as an obstacle to human progress more than anything else—are found wanting. The study takes seriously the role of traditional healing and important things are learned as a result. A complex interplay of spirituality and culture is what turns up when an effort is made to look more closely at health care in Africa. This is worth keeping in mind as thoughts turn to how health care works in an overall sense and its potential improvement in the future.

Who might want to read this book? The audience naturally begins with scholars in the interdisciplinary fields of African Studies, Religious Studies, and Health Studies. It is hoped that practitioners in the health sector, along with activists and policymakers, will also see value in this study.

Chapter outlines

Chapter 2 focuses on health services and religion in the African context to provide a foundation for the case studies in Chapters 3–5. Background knowledge is gleaned from the literature on the intersection of religion, health, and Africa. Patterns are identified, subsequently to be (dis)confirmed by the new evidence about Uganda, Mozambique, and Ethiopia. Theorizing about processes and outcomes regarding health, which includes a particular emphasis on women's health, comes next. Questions about the gathering of evidence—case selection, the profiling of the three states, and the methods of inquiry—are answered.

Chapter 3 on Uganda describes and analyzes how religion affects the provision and consumption of health services in that country. This chapter unfolds in the following sections. The first section conveys the political, economic, health, and religious contexts of the preceding research questions. Second, existing research on religion and health care in Uganda is summarized. The third section includes evidence. Interview material is organized into five subsections corresponding to: (1) the general importance of religion; (2) religion and health provision; (3) religion and health-seeking behavior; (4) traditional and spiritual healing; and (5) an evaluation of the role of religion in health care. A sixth subsection focuses on outcomes. Fourth, evidence about religious determinants of health in terms of processes (ie conveyed by interviewees) and outcomes (ie in the context of the MDGs) is assessed. The fifth and final section offers conclusions. The same steps are carried out in Chapters 4 and 5 on Mozambique and Ethiopia, respectively.

Chapter 6 conveys the findings from the three case studies in respective stages. First, it describes the role of religion in health care in terms of processes. What connections emerge in each state regarding the role of religion in the provision and seeking of health? The second stage, with a focus on the MDGs, is about outcomes. To what extent does religion contribute positively versus negatively to health care in each state? A third and final stage summarizes the chapter's insights.

Chapter 7 sums up what has been learned about the role of religion in the provision and consumption of health care in Uganda, Mozambique, and Ethiopia. The two basic questions motivating this study are answered to at least some degree: how does religion matter (1) within the SDOH frame of reference and (2) with regard to outcomes? Implications for the respective concepts of Africa, health, and religion, along with the interdisciplinary fields of African Studies, Health Studies, and Religious Studies, are identified. The chapter concludes with ideas for future research.

2

Background knowledge, theorizing, and evidence

Overview

This chapter explores the nexus of religion and health care, and serves as a foundation for the case studies that ensue in Chapters 3–5. Several things stand out by the time this chapter is completed. While individual items are quite good, the academic literature on religion and health care in relation to Africa is relatively limited in size. The work that does exist, however, is sufficient to establish that health care is regarded in a holistic way by Africans. The spiritual and physical worlds are intertwined. It therefore makes sense to take as a point of departure, theoretically speaking, a perspective offered by the Social Determinants of Health. This outlook on health is comprehensive and, as further chapters unfold, seems quite in line with the reality of at least the three states included in this volume and, in all likelihood, many more of those in Africa. The states covered—Uganda, Mozambique, and Ethiopia—are majority Christian and located in East Africa. Limitations related to the preceding sample are acknowledged. Given the holistic nature of health in the three states, interviews are regarded as essential to understanding both provision and consumption. This method of data gathering is implemented for all three cases.

Work begins with an exploration of background knowledge. What patterns can be identified already regarding the role of religion in health within Africa, the most challenged among the continents in terms of development across the board? This exercise is followed by theorizing from the perspective of the Social Determinants of Health, within which an emphasis on women's health will be applied to processes and outcomes. A discussion of evidence then follows. Case selection, the basic profiling of the countries along the most relevant dimensions, and methods are covered in that section. The final section sums up the contributions of the chapter.

Religion and health in Africa: background knowledge

Given the vast literature available through African Studies, Health Studies, and Religious Studies, collectively speaking, the review of background knowledge concentrates on items that combine these interests. Figure 2.1 conveys the scope of this review through its centroid—the intersection set of the three interdisciplinary fields. The key to Figure 2.1 provides a few examples in each instance for the seven sets of studies: those related to each interdisciplinary field (Religious Studies—I; African Studies—II; Health Studies—III), two-

Figure 2.1: African studies, religious studies, and health studies

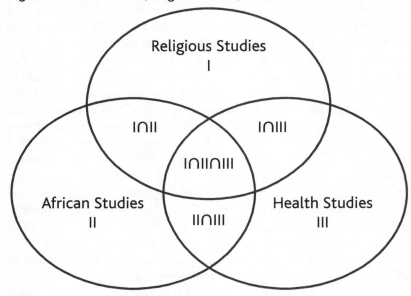

Key to Figure 2.1:

I: Turner (1981); Byrne (1988); Hatzopoulos and Petito (2003); Fox and Sandler (2004); Sharma (2005); Alles (2008, 2010); Fox (2008); Hassner (2009, 2012, 2016); Hoffman (2010); Moyser (2010); Sharpe (2010); Wolffe (2010); Haynes (2013); Malley (2013); Neusner (2013); Vernoff (2013)

II: Kisangani (1997, 2012); Pinkey (2001); Markakis (2011); Menkhaus (2014); African Studies Association (2016); Quinn (2016)

III: Becker (1974); Tatalovich (1997); Maioni (1998); Haussman (2005); Huber et al (2011); Suzuki (2015); Boyd-Judson and James (2014); Krishnamani (2015b)

I ∩ II: Mtibi (1969); Turner (1981, 1988); Ranger (1988); Chitando (2005); Kumar (2006); Asante and Mazama (2009)

I ∩ III: Ranger (1988); Cochrane (2006); Chand and Patterson (2007); Trinitapoli and Weinreb (2012); Hönke and Thauer (2014)

II ∩ III: Starr (1982); Vogel (1993); Parkhurst (2002); Natala (2006); Sama and Nguyen (2008); Cooke (2009); Richard et al (2011); Birhanu et al (2012); Callaghan-Koru et al (2013); Moftah (2014); Durr (2015); Linke et al (2015, forthcoming); Gros (2016); Deneulin and Zampini-Davies (2017)

I ∩ II ∩ III: The contents of the literature review from this chapter, collectively speaking, would appear in this subset.

way intersections (I ∩ II, I ∩ II, II ∩ III), and the three-way intersection (I ∩ II ∩ III). While studies from other areas in the figure will also be referenced in the analysis as appropriate, the review that follows incorporates the items that focus on the role of religion in health for Africa—the three-way intersection set.

Research intersecting on Africa, health, and religion is organized into the subject areas that follow. In terms of beliefs held by *consumers* of health, it will become apparent that holism is the norm. With regard to *producers* of health from the religious sphere—Faith-Inspired Institutions—the major topic areas covered by the literature are: (1) market share; (2) comparative advantage; (3) service to the poor and concentration on HIV/AIDS; and (4) challenges to success.

Consider how health care is *consumed* in Africa. References to the connection of physical and spiritual health among Africans are legion (Cochrane et al 2012: 130). In the African context, "the health sciences increasingly recognize that health is a life-span phenomenon in which access to specific medical services forms a small fraction of what determines the quality of health life along the way" and the strengths of congregations are "visible in African villages" (Gunderson and Cochrane 2012: 44, 45). "Africans," Gros (2016: 58) adds, had grasped the "holistic nature of health" before the World Health Organization defined it comprehensively. In a word, health-seeking Africans are holists. This trait, in turn, opens the door to influence from belief systems, notably, religion, among consumers of health care.

Holistic thinking among Africans comes through in any number of empirical, country-specific studies as well, with a few examples provided here. Olupona (2004) investigates divination and healing among the Yoruba in South-Western Nigeria. "As in most African groups," Olupona (2004: 111) asserts, "Yoruba theories of sickness and disease are connected to the construction of the world and social and cultural life." While Western medicine may be tried first, "if the illness persists, divination is a credible option" (Olupona 2004: 112). A priority on treating the whole person is clearly embedded within these observations about health-seeking behavior. Assertions from Obinna (2012) about indigenous healers in Amasiri, Nigeria, parallel those just outlined. "Indigenous healing," observes Obinna (2012: 135), "reveals a process in which the healer, client, and the social and cosmological order of the Amasiri interact to bring about meaningful, desired results of healing to individuals, groups, or community." Within the Amisiri community, "indigenous healers serve not only as healers but also as consultants on family, village, and clan matters" (Obinna 2012: 135). These patterns are in line with a holistic view of health among those involved. So, too, are the religious aspects in a study by Westerlund (2006) of disease etiologies among five African peoples. Over the course of a century, a shift is evident from an emphasis on the role of spirits *per se* to humans such as witches (Westerlund 2006: 189–208).

Attention now shifts from how health care is consumed to how it is *produced*. One of the ongoing controversies about faith-based institutions concerns accurate assessment regarding their share of the health-care market. Realistic descriptions of their size and power have been difficult to reach because "barely any of the evidence is measured using the same indicator or measure" and Faith-Inspired Institutions tend to fall into gray areas as they are often engaged in more than faith-based enterprises and frequently partner with their government or other non-governmental organizations (NGOs) (Olivier and Wodon 2012d: 11, 12). For example, health facilities in various states are co-owned by Faith-Inspired Institutions and government providers (Olivier and Wodon 2012d: 12). Several factors may lead, in particular, to *over*estimation of the market share for Faith-Based Organizations: provision of services by facilities other than hospitals; missing data on private non-religious facilities; and exclusion of some providers from statistics (Olivier and Wodon 2012d: 15). *Under*estimation is also possible "because some faith-inspired facilities may have been considered by households as public facilities given that in many districts, faith-inspired hospitals serve as district hospitals" (Olivier et al 2012d: 130). In sum, the estimated market share for Faith-Based Organizations is quite sensitive to the type of metric used—much higher for hospital beds or formal facilities as opposed to household surveys (Olivier and Wodon 2012d: 17, 20, 21).

Olivier et al (2012a: 15), in search of a more accurate assessment of market share, assessed "the availability of data identifying faith-inspired health providers in the main multi-purpose surveys implemented in approximately 30 African countries." When divided into quintiles, the market shares for faith-inspired facilities look similar to those of public facilities (Olivier et al 2012a: 14). Faith-Inspired Institutions do reveal a slightly higher market share among the very poor and serve those worst off more than other non-state, non-religious facilities-based providers (Olivier et al 2012a: 18, 20). To a certain extent, Faith-Inspired Institutions compete for market share but are largely complementary to state-based health care. Wodon et al (2012: 36), on the basis of their data, infer a lower market share for Faith-Based Organizations than previously believed based on the provision of treatment for various maladies, such as a fever or cough.

What about the question of comparative advantage? Olivier and Wodon (2012f: 1; see also 2012e) assert that claims for comparative advantage regarding Faith-Inspired Institutions' health care *per se* are "poorly evidenced." Specific information is available from a survey of Burundi, Mali, Senegal, Republic of Congo, and Ghana: Faith-Based Organizations do not have a significant comparative advantage versus private secular and public facilities regarding waiting times (Tsimpo and Wodon 2012: 83). In fairness, however, Faith-Inspired Institutions are blocked by resource limitations from serving the poor more than others do (Tsimpo and Wodon 2012: 89). Based on interviews and quantitative data from Ghana, the research team of Shojo et al (2012: 80) report that levels of satisfaction are similar for public and Faith-Inspired Institutions' facilities.

Some evidence exists, however, that Faith-Inspired Institutions engender greater levels of trust and satisfaction among users. Based on fieldwork in the West African state of Burkina Faso, the research team of Gemignani and Wodon (2012: 60, 61) enumerate the following specific advantages noted by patients regarding Faith-Inspired Institutions, over and above high satisfaction with care: lower treatment costs; good relationships between personnel and patients; and overall quality of care. Respondents at Christian and Islamic clinics in Burkina Faso identified a wide range of advantages associated with Faith-Based Organizations: general improvements in health care due to better attendance; improved antenatal and postnatal care; the availability of nutritional programs; and stronger attention by providers to social and economic issues (Gemignani and Wodon 2012: 64). Gemignani and Wodon (2012: 66) also made the interesting observation that the work of Faith-Inspired Institutions "helps to reduce barriers faced by women in accessing care."

Evidence from household surveys in Burundi, Ghana, Mali, Niger, Republic of Congo, and Senegal "suggests that FIIs [Faith-Inspired Institutions] do appear to enjoy higher satisfaction rates than public facilities" (Olivier et al 2012b: 15). Moreover, respondents to the surveys noted that willingness to pray with patients and the provision of compassionate care stood out as positive traits for Faith-Based Organizations (Olivier et al 2012b: 23, 25). Along similar lines, a study of the Democratic Republic of the Congo revealed considerable goodwill from government, representative, and other groups toward Christian religious entities in the context of health-care provision. In particular, the level of trust stood out in facilitating effective partnerships between Christian Faith-Inspired Institutions, on the one hand, and donors, on the other (Olivier and Haddad 2012: 179, 180).

Olivier and Wodon (2012b: 46), in an overall sense, warn against any broad statements about comparative (dis)advantage for Faith-Inspired Institutions. The truth is likely that Faith-Based Organizations are advantaged in some ways and disadvantaged in others.

As would be understood from the Social Determinants of Health approach, poverty and governmental unwillingness to allocate proper funding are underlying reasons for many health challenges in Africa. One very pernicious feature is the degree of control over policy by state elites, which creates a "vicious cycle" in favor of supporters (Quinn 2016: 101). In other words, areas favoring the opposition in a given African state can be expected to suffer in comparison to those that are pro-government when it comes to public services such as health care (Quinn 2016: 100–101, 175).

Faith-Inspired Institutions play a special role in serving the poor. Health-care providers are in chronically short supply (Dielman et al 2012: 101; see also Dimmock et al 2012: 84). With a focus on Nairobi, Kenya, the research team of Blevins et al (2012) used mapping technology to study the especially impoverished Mukuru network of villages. In this setting, community health assets do not have a formal home. Instead, religious organizations provide the majority of the structure (Blevins et al 2012: 94). A study of Ghana reveals the key role of the Catholic Church in provision—all of those who live in a given area may benefit from its health services (Coulombe and Wodon 2012a: 73, 2012b). A survey of Salvation Army health programs in more than 30 countries sees value in health institutions providing "a hub for a web of relationships with others including place of worship and households" (Pallant 2012: 91). An approach that incorporates Faith-Inspired Institutions in an institutional network is most promising, according to Pallant (2012: 95), with regard to improving the health of the poorest people. A study of Burkina Faso concurs, with Faith-Based Organizations singled out for reducing the costs of health care in order to reach very poor members of society (Gemignani et al 2012: 110, 118).[1] In addition, the work of Bulembu Ministries, which includes assistance to abandoned children, stands out in this context (Harron 2015: 10).

---

[1]　Numerous studies reaffirm the value of partnerships at the local level, which frequently involve Faith-Based Organizations, to enhance the legitimacy of health-care efforts. These partnerships facilitate health services to the most marginalized and vulnerable communities (Karam 2012; Olivier and Haddad 2012; Beisheim et al 2014; Hönke and Thauer 2014; Schäferhoff 2014).

Faith-Inspired Institutions play a significant ongoing role in the fight against HIV/AIDS (Agadjanian 2012; Boulenger et al 2012; Harron 2015). Foster et al (2012: 118, 120) report that virtually all churches in Zimbabwe have implemented HIV-related activities and religious organizations continue to collaborate within a network that is leading to "improved health outcomes." With a focus on Zambia and Lesotho, the research team of Olivier, Cochrane, and De Gruchy (2012c: 56, 57) carried out a mapping of religious entities. Faith-Inspired Institutions play a major role in the fight against HIV/AIDS at a local level and "leading intangibles are spiritual encouragement, knowledge giving and moral formation" (Toefy 2009: 248). The study concludes that greater engagement of governments with religious entities that provide health would be to the benefit of all (Olivier et al 2012c: 57). A study of 85 congregations in villages from rural Malawi confirms that religious organizations are active in that state as well (Trinitapoli 2006: 257). It is interesting to note that opposition among religious leaders to the use of condoms is not monolithic (Trinitapoli 2006: 262). Programs vary from one church to another, but the overall conclusion is that religious leaders in rural Malawi "promote conservative messages about sexual behavior and HIV risk" (Trinitapoli 2006) through sermons and represent an untapped resource for working against the spread of HIV. Moreover, the clergy do not stigmatize those with the affliction (Trinitapoli 2006: 267, 268).

Challenges are also identified in the academic literature about health provision in Africa. Faith-Based Organizations have some common problems, most notably, limited resources (Giusti no date; Dimmock et al 2012: 84; Gemignani and Wodon 2012: 67). More specifically, Faith-Inspired Institutions face difficulties with cost–recovery mechanisms (Olivier et al 2012a: 21). They also have implicitly normative or moral obligations to treat those who cannot pay.

Other problems pertain to the religious mission of Faith-Based Organizations in conjunction with their larger setting in society and connection with government. In Burkina Faso, for instance, it is difficult for faith-based health centers to promote the use of family planning and, at the same time, there is always the risk of accusations about proselytizing (Gemignani and Wodon 2012: 67). Christian facilities, in various places, struggle to maintain their mission while confronting the tensions caused by integration with the public sector (Dimmock et al 2012: 85; Olivier et al 2012a: 21). Olivier and Wodon (2012a: 149) offer a long list of problems faced by Faith-Inspired Institutions along those lines, notably, in relation to obtaining HIV/AIDS resources: secular governments do not want to fund them;

funders fear that resources might be used for proselytism; there is a historic distrust of government and international funding processes; and there is a lack of capacity for dealing with complex funding proposals and evaluations.

Looking back on the academic literature, points of consensus emerge that provide an intellectual context for this study as it unfolds. Africans, as consumers of health care, tend toward a holistic point of view. The physical and spiritual worlds are believed to operate together rather than in isolation. This opens the door to both faith-based provision of modern health care and traditional healing. With regard to faith-based providers, there is some degree of controversy over exact market shares but no disagreement about basic significance within the full network of health care. Comparative advantage for Faith-Inspired Institutions is not confirmed, and to the extent that it operates, it probably does so in a complicated and highly contextualized manner. A clearer picture emerges from the academic literature on service to the poor and coping with HIV/AIDS: faith-based providers are active and effective in those areas. Finally, with regard to problem areas for religious providers of health care, the lack of resources and difficulties in coordinating with the public sector stand out.

Theorizing

How do the religious beliefs of Africans affect the understanding, access, and delivery of health and health care? To answer this question, the point of departure will be the Social Determinants of Health frame of reference. Religion will be viewed as a categorical independent variable defined via belief system: (1) Africans are placed into different religious categories; and (2) beliefs in categories such as Christian, Muslim, African Traditional Religion, Syncretistic, and secular are assessed in terms of how they affect understanding of health. How health is understood, in turn, is anticipated to impact upon health-seeking behavior. This behavior is further broken down by demand (understood and accessed) and supply (secular versus religious provision). In other words, Africans are conceptualized as rational actors, with the goal of health being pursued under conditions that very frequently include both spiritual and physical dimensions.

Within the Social Determinants of Health framework, both processes and outcomes are investigated. The nature of the provider, health-seeking behavior among consumers, and the influence of religion collectively constitute the processes. Outcomes are assessed in terms of standard benchmarks, the Millennium Development Goals. As observed in Chapter 1, the eight Millennium Development Goals are intertwined and work well in measuring health outcomes in a comprehensive way. Along those lines, recall the World Health Organization's definition of health: "a state of complete physical, mental and social well-being and not merely the absence of disease or infirmity." The wide range of indicators included in the Millennium Development Goals—everything from education to combating disease—is in line with that definition.

From a social-scientific standpoint, given the presence of presumed independent and dependent variables, the articulation of a conceptual model of the impact of religion on seeking and providing health would seem like the natural next step. Rather than directional propositions, however, the preference here is for exploratory research that identifies associations for intensive, data-based scrutiny when resources become more fully available. Given the basis of this project in Religious Studies, African Studies, and Health Studies, as described earlier, the theoretical foundation will be interdisciplinary. Concepts from economic theory—supply and demand—have already been mentioned. In addition, gender-oriented analysis will be brought to bear on both process and outcomes.

These choices—an economic model of provision and consumption of health care, along with a gender-related emphasis for interpretation—provide a structure for analysis but not a Procrustean bed. Rigorously stated propositions, by contrast, might be regarded as a goal for future research rather than a guiding force as the pages of this book unfold. This inductive approach seems justified and even prudent given the preceding discussion of concept formation. Consider, along so many dimensions, the diversity of Africa. The relatively scarce collection of pan-African studies on religion and health care provide a starting point rather than a massive database from within which to borrow and apply well-tested hypotheses. Indeed, the research on religion and health care in Africa, reviewed a moment ago, focuses on Faith-Based Organizations along the following dimensions: market share; comparative advantage; service to the poor and coping with HIV/AIDS; and challenges to success. It is impossible to glean from that work with any specificity directional hypotheses that pertain to the role of religion in the provision and consumption of health, especially at an individual level.

Intuition does favor two ideas, if not formally stated propositions. First, given the rise of religion around the world (aside from a few exceptional locations), it is likely that faith will matter significantly vis-a-vis health care in terms of both provision and consumption.

This should be especially true in African states where demand exceeds supply under conditions of deprivation that represent the norm. Second, persistent poverty in Africa also suggests that gender-related analysis will prove relevant before all is said and done because of its likely unequal impact via the health system. The analysis is guided by these ideas, which, in turn, may eventually combine to produce propositions for more rigorous assessment as case studies accumulate and data become available.

Two points of qualification should be offered with regard to the analysis carried out in this book. One aspect concerns religious processes, while the other focuses on the nature of the sample included for study.

First, religious processes can be significant in influencing the decisions that people make about important matters such as seeking health care. Much value certainly would exist in probing, for instance, religious doctrines and their implementation within a given church in the effort to explain what people are trying to do about their health. This topic is beyond the scope of the present study and will be addressed briefly in Chapter 7 as a priority for future research.

Second, the three states included in the book are not here because of any rigorous selection process. Instead, given difficulties attached to the subject matter—religion (a highly sensitive topic) in the context of Africa (a challenging location in terms of logistics)—the states that appear in this study should be regarded as a convenience sample. Capabilities and limitations of the team of co-authors, along with the need for support on the ground from the Institute for Global Health at the University of Southern California (USC), determined the choice of the three states covered in this book. In addition, the sheer number of cases could not be increased, at least for the short- to -medium term purposes of a book-length study, due to resource constraints in an overall sense.

Evidence

This section will answer questions about the gathering of evidence. The issues, respectively, concern case selection, profiling the three states included in this study to gain a sense of their representativeness, and methods.

With so many states in Africa, what value exists in studying just three of them? An excellent study of health care in Africa—coincidentally, one that also includes exactly three cases—took up this point quite recently. "On the practical side," observes Gros (2016: 17), "no one should expect one researcher to 'case study' fifty-five countries, unless the research spans an entire lifetime, and even that might not be enough (resources matter, too)." What makes more sense is to be quite careful about what is inferred from a small "N" such as three. The present study might properly be viewed as one in search of depth rather than breadth. The forthcoming interview-based evidence from Uganda, Mozambique, and Ethiopia will be most valuable in terms of generating rather than confirming ideas with regard to any domain beyond the boundaries of those states.

Table 2.1 profiles Uganda, Mozambique, and Ethiopia along selected dimensions, with the US as the quasi-hegemonic system leader added for some points of comparison. The table's contents reveal similarity across some dimensions, with degrees of uniqueness as well. Ethiopia and Mozambique are much greater than Uganda in geographic expanse. Ethiopia stands alone in terms of population, being much larger than the other two states. The age distribution is very young across all three countries. Standard of living is relatively close, ranging from USD1,200 to USD1,500 in gross domestic product (GDP) per capita, while Ethiopia lags very far behind in literacy. Note that the US is ahead by orders of magnitude with regard to per capita income and literacy.

Figures for the representation of women in national parliaments are relatively high by standards for developing states, with 28% of the Ugandan Parliament as the minimum in the table. Oddly enough, the US is at the low end for this indicator.

All three states feature Christian majorities, with Mozambique at the low end with 52%. This is a point in common with the US, where Christians are at 59%. As acknowledged earlier, the research does not therefore include a Muslim-majority state. Efforts to obtain interviews with Muslim academics and Faith-Based Organizations, however, proved to be successful. Thus, at least some insight can be obtained into how provision and consumption of health care works within the context of Islam. Further research that would focus on Muslim-majority states is discussed a bit further as a research priority in Chapter 7.

With regard to the Millennium Development Goals, there are encouraging percentage changes to observe in Table 2.1 for the African states. (As expected, the numbers for the US are much better across the board.) Child mortality (Goal 4) and maternal mortality (Goal 5) are down at least 60% and 54%, respectively, from 1990 across the three states up to 2012/2013. With regard to mortality from infectious diseases (Goal 6), the pattern is also favorable. For HIV/AIDS, malaria, and tuberculosis, only Mozambique, for HIV/AIDS, shows an increase.

Table 2.1: Selected indicators for Uganda, Mozambique, and Ethiopia

Country	Uganda	Mozambique	Ethiopia	USA
Size (sq km)[a]	241,038	799,380	1,104,300	9,833,517
Population[a]	35,918,915	24,692,144	90,633,458	323,995,528
Median age[a]	15.5	16.9	17.6	37.9
Per capita GDP USD[a]	1,500	1,200	1,300	57,300
Literacy rate (percentage 15 and older who read and write)[a]	73.2	56.1	39	97.9
Representation of women (%)[d]	28	40	35	20
Religious affiliation (by percentage and of total)[b]	**Christians 84** (Extended Protestants 42 [Anglicans 37; Pentacostals 3; Mainline Protestants 2] Catholics 40; Orthodox 1) **Muslims 12** (Sunni 10; Other 2) **Animist 2**	**Christians 52** (Catholics 30; Extended Protestants 19 [Pentacostals 11; Mainline Protestants 7; Anglicans 1]; Orthodox 3) **Muslims 18** (Sunni 18) **Animist 29**	**Christians 63** (Orthodox 42; Extended Protestants 21 [Mainline Protestants 18; Pentacostals 3]; Catholics 1) **Muslims 34** (Sunni 33; Other 1) **Animist 2**	**Christians 59** (Extended Protestants 30 [Anglicans 25; Pentacostals 25]; Catholics 23; Orthodox 2) **Muslims 1** **Animist < 1**

Table 2.2: Social indicators in the three nations

Country	MDG2—Net enrolment ratio in primary education (enrollees per 100 children)	MDG4—Child mortality per 1,000 live births[c]	MDG5a—Maternal mortality per 1,000 live births[c]	MDG5b—Current contraceptive use among married women 15–49 years old, any method, %	MDG6—Mortality from infectious diseases per 100,000 inhabitants[c]	Percentage of funds to health sector, average for 2007–2011
Uganda	2009 2013 Δ% 91.4 91.6 0	1990 2000 2012 Δ% 178 147 69 −61	1990 2000 2013 Δ% 780 650 360 −54	1995 2005 2014 Δ% 14.8 19.7 27.2 12.4	2000 2012 HIV/AIDS 4094 380 Malaria 47470 175 TB 4262 175	10.4
Mozambique	1990 2013 Δ% 44 87.6 99	1990 2000 2012 Δ% 233 166 90 −61	1990 2000 2013 Δ% 1300 870 480 −63	1997 2004 2011 Δ% 5.6 25.5 11.6 6	2000 2012 HIV/AIDS 4508 6169 Malaria --- 7714 TB 701 553	9.99
Ethiopia	1994 2006 Δ% 19.2 66.1 244	1990 2000 2012 Δ% 204 146 68 −67	1990 2000 2013 Δ% 1400 990 420 −70	1997 2005 2014 Δ% 3.3 14.7 34.2 30.9	2000 2012 HIV/AIDS 1912 827 Malaria --- 4132 TB 429 224	13.42
USA	1990 2000 2013 Δ% 97.2 96.6 92.4 −5	1990 2000 2012 Δ% 11.2 8.4 7.1 −37	1990 2000 2013 Δ% 12 12 14 17	1990 2002 2010 Δ% 70.7 72.8 76.4 5.7	2000 2012 HIV/AIDS - - - - - Malaria - - - - - - TB 0.3 0.2	*

Note: * A percentage estimate for the US is left blank for now because of ongoing efforts to repeal and replace the Affordable Care Act. Percentage change is between first and last data point for each category. MDG = Millennium Development Goal; TB = tuberculosis.

Sources: [a] CIA World Factbook (2014) (see: https://www.cia.gov/library/publications/the-world-factbook/geos/et.html); [b] Brown and James (2015) (all data are from 2010); [c] Gros (2016: 139, 141, 142–143); [d] Inter-Parliamentary Union (2016).

The overall pattern for health is toward improvement in percentage terms but, importantly, much work remains because the figures had previously been quite unimpressive coming into the new millennium.

With regard to the percentage of funds going to health care, the governments of Uganda and Mozambique are close together—a bit above and below 10%. Ethiopia, the poorest of the three states, comes in at 13.42%.

From Table 2.1, a picture emerges of Uganda, Mozambique, and Ethiopia as largely representative of African states and fundamentally different from the US. This is not meant to say that the collection of three states covered in this volume is representative of Africa in the rigorous sense of something like a stratified cluster analysis from survey research. Instead, these states are sufficiently diverse for the purposes of probing the plausibility of intuition about religion as a significant element of the Social Determinants of Health on the African continent. The generation rather than testing of ideas is appropriate with a sample of this kind.

With regard to methods, this study is based on interviews in conjunction with primary and secondary research. The interviewees included Faith-Inspired Institutions, government officials, and academics with research interests in health care. In terms of location, the interviews tilt toward urban areas, but at least some took place in a rural setting. Some interviewees either gave their names ahead of time or offered that information at the time of the meeting. For ethical reasons, no interviewee is identified by name in this book because of safety considerations that either exist already or might arise in the future.

While statistics play a role in this project, and the Millennium Development Goals are certainly primarily measured with numbers, no quantitative analysis in the rigorous sense appears. Olivier and Wodon (2012a: 2), in reflecting upon studies focusing on Africa and health, offer a thoughtful summing up of differences involving quantitative versus qualitative approaches:

> Mapping studies based on "hard" evidence (such as health facilities surveys) are usually valued more highly at a policy level than the "softer" approaches which might seek to understand how individuals and communities perceive or relate to the facilities and assets being mapped. But "softer" approaches tend to result in more nuanced layers of evidence and results, which may also be beneficial. Choosing the right mapping approach depends on the objective sought.

The present study leans toward the soft end of the continuum of approaches, with two basic points of justification. One is the focus on Africa, a region in which statistical data are most difficult to collect and even hard to fully trust when available. The other point to consider is the central role of religion in the subject matter of this project. Olivier and Wodon (2012a) affirm that a softer approach—meaning one based on how people perceive things—can have value. With the faith-based provision and consumption of health care as a basic concern, it makes sense to give pride of place to reflections from people about their opportunities and choices.

Interviews took place in a semi-structured format. This is a standard approach toward interviewing experts such as health-care professionals, administrators, and the like.[2] Whenever possible, interviewees received an email message ahead of time that provided a basic agenda of interest and tentative questions. This is appropriate because experts, all other things being equal, respond best when given some flexibility in providing information. An excessive amount of structure, in other words, can be offensive to someone who believes that they have superior command of the specific subject matter at hand. Experiences throughout the interviews conducted for this project reaffirmed that intuition, which is based on a wide range of prior studies.

Outcomes will be assessed via figures for the Millennium Development Goals. These goals "represent an unprecedented global consensus about measures to reduce poverty" (Waage et al 2010: 991) and therefore set compelling priorities for the evaluation of state performance. To link processes with outcomes directly would be challenging. However, at the very least, inferences can be made in terms of direction. In other words, do the processes revealed by interviews tend to point toward or away from improvement in Millennium Development Goals?

Moving Forward

Background knowledge reveals that religion matters for the production and consumption of health in Africa. Research is of high quality but relatively low quantity, which, in turn, impacts upon this study's approach toward theorizing. Rather than highly specific, directional hypotheses, research is guided by intuition about the supply of and demand for health care, along with an emphasis on women's health, for interpretation.

---

[2]   For a detailed treatment of implementation vis-a-vis semi-structured interviews, see Huang and James (2014).

With over 50 states in Africa and just three included in this study, the work is better viewed as an exercise in the generation rather than testing of ideas anyway. Research in subsequent chapters on Uganda, Mozambique, and Ethiopia will search for patterns and meaning with respect to the role of religion in the provision and consumption of health.

3

Uganda

Overview

This chapter focuses on religion and the Social Determinants of Health in Uganda, a low-income, developing country with a complex history that includes independent African kingdoms, British colonial rule, and independence since 1962. The two basic questions from Chapter 1 will be answered to varying degrees: "How does religion contribute to the Social Determinants of Health?"; and "What is its connection to outcomes?"

This chapter, to foreshadow its contributions, begins with an overall sense of Uganda as a poor state with a mixed and frequently unsuccessful performance from its government. With regard to health care, efforts toward planning exist but the government either lacks or fails to provide sufficient resources to produce good outcomes across the board. For example, state-created Village Health Teams have led to some improvements but not all regions possess this resource and the overall level of funding is simply inadequate to meet public needs. This ongoing feature of life in Uganda opens the door to faith-based provision. Ugandans, on the whole, are quite religious and efforts from Faith-Based Organizations to offer health services are well received. Traditional healing finds a place alongside modern medicine, with unscientific practices linked to witchcraft receding into the background but not disappearing altogether. Religious institutions have positive effects overall but impact to some degree in a negative way on women's health as assessed on the basis of the Millennium Development Goals (MDGs). In sum, the chapter will reveal that religion plays an essential role in Uganda for both the provision and consumption of health care.

Located in Eastern Africa, the Republic of Uganda is slightly smaller than the American state of Oregon. Uganda is a landlocked state bordered by Rwanda, the Democratic Republic of Congo (DRC), South Sudan, and Kenya. Uganda also shares a border with Tanzania along Lake Victoria and has a fast-growing population of about 37 million people, which is a bit larger than the American state of California. The capital and largest city in Uganda is Kampala, located near Lake Victoria (CIA World Factbook 2016).

Uganda is ethno-linguistically diverse, with 41 languages (Ethnologue 2016a). English is the official language in the country, though Ganda (or Luganda) is also used for wider communication. Swahili (or Kiswahili) is the national language of Uganda, though Luganda is spoken as a lingua franca in Buganda.[1]

Since independence, Uganda has had an ongoing struggle with persistent poverty. According to United Nations (UN) data, in 2012 (the most recent year for which information is available), 37.8% of the population lived on less than USD1.25 per day (calculated in terms of purchasing power parity). While down significantly from the 71.9% of the population living on less than USD1.25 in 1992, well over one third of Ugandans continue to face endemic poverty and hunger. Furthermore, wealth in the country is unevenly distributed—according to the World Bank, Uganda had a Gini coefficient[2] of 45 in 2012.

Primary research reported in this chapter pertains to contemporary Uganda, which continues on the path to full development. Two research teams with personnel from universities in the US, USC and Pepperdine University, conducted interviews in and around Kampala during February/March 2012 and January 2013.[3] Interviews included government officials, politicians, academics, and non-governmental organization (NGO) employees. Contacts from USC's Institute for Global Health, notably, the public health consultant Robert Ssebugwawo, greatly facilitated access to a wide range of well-informed interviewees. A list of interviews, and dates, appears in the Appendix (see p 195).

Available research on how health care is linked to religion in Uganda is of high quality, but it is relatively limited and tends to be reported at the national level. The intended contribution for this resource is focused at the individual level to assess conventional wisdom and inform policy by adding depth to complement existing breadth. The

---

[1] Differences between national and official languages are as follows: "it generally appears that the 'official' language of a country is the one in which the laws of the country are made and publicized, whereas the 'national' language is the one which is used, more often orally, in parliament, administration, mass-media, primary education and literacy campaigns; but laws do not have to be passed nor published in them. National languages are also those which were used by the broad masses during their anti-colonial struggle and which enjoyed a sufficient amount of literacy and literary tradition" (Lodhi 1993: 81).

[2] The Gini coefficient is a measurement of income inequality in a country.

[3] The teams consisted of Laura Ferguson, Patrick James, and Robert Lloyd (in 2012) and Nuvjote Hundal, Patrick James, Robert Lloyd, and Heather Wipfli (in 2013). The multi-person teams included, in each instance, expertise on religion, health care, and Africa in general.

current chapter might be viewed as a sequel to Schmid et al (2008), an outstanding evaluation of how religion and health care are related to each other in Uganda.[4]

This chapter unfolds in four additional sections. The first section conveys the political, social, economic, health-care, and religious context of Uganda to frame the discussion. The second section summarizes existing research on religion and health care in Uganda. The third section, on faith-based health provision and behavior, includes interview material on processes organized into subsections corresponding to: (1) the general importance of religion; (2) religion and health provision; (3) religion and health-seeking behavior; (4) traditional and spiritual healing; and (5) the evaluation of the role of religion in health care. A further subsection covers outcomes with regard to the MDGs. The fourth and final section passes along conclusions.

Context

While post-colonial political turmoil has characterized its history, Uganda has emerged into a generally stable republic (lack of government control over the north would be the main exception). The Ugandan government is composed of three branches: executive, legislative, and judicial. The politics of contemporary Uganda took shape when Yoweri Kaguta Museveni, head of the National Resistance Army, led a successful overthrow of the short-lived Okello military government in 1986 (Schmid et al 2008: 126). Museveni and the National Resistance Army enjoyed genuine widespread popular support during their insurgency, which led them to accomplish a first in Africa: having an insurgent army successfully capture and retain power, as opposed to coming to power via palace coup (Pinkney 2001: 162–163). Museveni rechristened the National Resistance Army as the National Resistance Movement political party, which became the dominant force in Ugandan politics. Over time, the National Resistance Movement effectively fused itself with state institutions, and both Parliament and the judiciary are seen as not being independent (Lugalambi et al 2010).

---

[4]   Methods used in combination by Schmid et al (2008) for three country case studies, including Uganda, are as follows: 10 key informant interviews that included representatives of the public health sector, some religious leaders, academics, and practitioners; three or four focus group discussions of 10 people per country, with representatives of identified faith-based health services; and questionnaires distributed to the same Faith-Based Organizations—about 25 per country.

In 2013, 57% of Ugandans surveyed believed that Parliament was corrupt and 79% believed the judiciary to be corrupt (Transparency International 2013; Lugalambi et al 2010).

Uganda is democratic "on paper" and has instituted a regime of holding multiparty elections. However, with a score of 5.5, it is rated as "not free" by Freedom House. Its leadership, at this time of writing, is in the habit of using the rest of the world as a scapegoat for health-care problems in Uganda. This tactic, which is intended to draw attention away from government shortcomings, impedes a sense of responsibility for addressing the persistent health-care challenges that face its people.

With a score of 2.5 on a 0–10 scale, Uganda does quite poorly on Transparency International's Corruption Perceptions Index; most misconduct takes place in the public sector and the procurement of goods and services is reputed to be especially abusive (Lugalambi et al 2010). Even when the government is willing to act, huge problems of capacity persist. For instance, the government decided in the 1990s to introduce sexual health education in the primary school curriculum (Shuey et al 1999: 412). However, follow-up studies routinely show that the program is having a limited impact due to the lack of effective teachers and other resources (Kinsman 2010). A World Bank study of learning in Uganda showed some elements of progress but also significant challenges in the school system (Najjumba et al. 2013). Accordingly, some have advocated for non-governmental actors, most notably, religious entities, to take on a larger role in the education and health sectors. Here, too, however, questions about training and capacity persist (Siu and Whyte 2009).

There are four main regions in Uganda: Central, Western, Eastern, and Northern. The regions are roughly the same size in terms of population. These regions are further divided into 111 districts and the city of Kampala. Table 3.1 presents selected data for religion by region. Christians are a majority across the board, with either Catholics or Anglicans as the plurality (or even majority) in a given region. The 2002 census reveals 12.1% of the population to be Muslim. The Central region recorded the highest Muslim proportion with 18.4%, followed closely by the Eastern region with 17%. At 4.6%, the Western region contains the lowest percentage of Muslim population.

Table 3.1: Religion by district for the population of Uganda (%)

Religion	Central	Eastern	Northern	Western	Uganda
Catholic	41.2	29.6	58.6	40.6	41.9
Anglican	31	43	23.1	45.2	35.9
Pentecostal	5.9	6.1	2.8	3.4	4.6
Muslim	18.4	17	7.6	4.5	12.1
Total region population	6,572,344	6,292,924	5,362,317	6,295,547	24,433,132

Note: District figures and smaller religious groups are excluded here.

Source: Government of Uganda (2002).

How, then, are government and religion connected with each other? Many governments seek to control religion—some are quite draconian in their approach (Fox 2008)—and the exercise of faith in Uganda has not been without interference from the state. During the time of Idi Amin (1971–1979), for example, the Nubian culture gained some ground and the brutal regime made conversion to Islam an attractive option from the standpoint of political advancement. The regime since then has been more benign. National holidays, such as Christmas Day, recognize the centrality of Christianity and Islam to life in Uganda.[5] State restrictions on religion, as reported in the authoritative compilation from Fox (2008: 282), are moderate in Uganda by world standards. All religious organizations must register with the government. Political parties with an exclusively religious membership are banned in Uganda and local governments frequently harass groups that appear to be cults (Fox 2008: 282).

While classified by the World Bank as a "low-income" country, Uganda possesses abundant natural and human resources. The country has experienced solid economic growth over the past decade. Policy impediments, however, block the rapid growth essential to reduce the country's still high poverty rate. Long-standing and deeply rooted poverty—now mostly in rural areas—is a great challenge in Uganda, particularly with regard to health. Life expectancy is 51.9 years and Uganda is ranked 157 out of 182 states on the United Nations Development Programme (UNDP) Human Development Index (Lugalambi et al 2010). "Poverty," as Natala (2006: 137) observes,

---

[5]   The full list of holidays includes Good Friday, Easter Sunday and Monday, Martyr's Day (Christian), Eid Al-Fitr, Eid Al-Adha, Christmas Day, and Boxing Day (World Trade Press n.d.: 4–6).

"is rated as the number one killer disease in Uganda" and affects the entire population "by lowering development." An annual 3.2% population increase puts pressure on agriculture, and, furthermore, energy shortages have slowed economic growth (Lugalambi et al 2010). Lagging rural development and limited poverty reduction are especially troubling for a state where agriculture accounts for about one third of gross domestic product (GDP) (Schmid et al 2008: 126).[6] Approximately 31% of the population lives on even less than a dollar per day (Lugalambi et al 2010). Transportation beyond relatively urbanized Kampala remains primitive; the road network is poorly maintained due to corruption and low investment.[7]

Consequences for health care from widespread poverty are quite evident in effective service provision: 85% of Ugandans are below the poverty line and "it therefore makes access to medical care difficult if not impossible brought about by inadequate medical service delivery which results in households using their meager incomes to fill the gap" (Natala 2006: 137–138). Maternal health is an especially challenging area. The country is demographically one of the fastest growing in the world, with approximately half the population being under 15 years of age. Uganda's fertility rate is high: 6.9 children, on average, for women who live through childbearing age (Natala 2006: 142). These numbers put great pressure on the medical infrastructure, with health centers not able to respond adequately and promptly (Schmid et al 2008: 127). The resulting maternal mortality rate is 310 per 100,000 live births and infant mortality is 76 per 1,000 live births (World Health Organization, cited in Tolchinsky 2013), compared to an average of 510 in sub-Saharan Africa as a whole. In all of this, the role of the Catholic Church represents something of a paradox: it is a major provider of health care but does not include family planning services.

Aside from health issues associated with pregnancy, most diseases causing mortality are communicable, though the burdens of non-communicable disease (stroke, heart disease, cancer, and respiratory disease) are increasing rapidly (Tolchinsky 2013). Approximately

---

[6]   Reasons enumerated by Natala (2006: 140) for sustained and even rising poverty are multifaceted and, taken together, quite challenging: "A) A slowdown in agricultural growth relative to non-agriculture sectors. B) A fall in agricultural prices reflecting unfavorable world market conditions. C) High fertility and mortality rates. D) Inefficiencies in targeting public expenditure towards poverty eradication. E) Social and cultural factors, particularly high consumption of alcohol, conflict and post-conflict effects."

[7]   Lugalambi et al (2010) also mention bad weather as a challenge to maintaining a road network—a matter obviously beyond state control.

1.2 million Ugandans live with HIV/AIDS—a predominantly heterosexually driven epidemic that remains a problem even with a decline from its peak of 18% in the 1990s (Kagimu et al 2012a: 17; 2012d: 286).

Uganda is sometimes cited as a global leader in HIV prevention, control, and management, but not without controversy. Uganda featured some valuable innovations, such as free voluntary testing centers in the 1990s. Emphasis has been on prevention rather than treatment, notably, with the "ABC" program founded upon *Abstinence* (A), along with *Be* Faithful (B), and *Condom* usage (C). Critics, however, have claimed that the HIV/AIDS statistics from Uganda are biased downward due to faulty data-gathering procedures (Parkhurst 2002). As a result, the jury remains out on Uganda's overall performance with respect to HIV/AIDS.

HIV/AIDS and war have taken their toll, of course, "but more easily cured killers like hunger, malaria, typhus, and sleeping sickness serve as the big culprits" (World Trade Press n.d.; see also Schmid et al 2008: 127). Data from Table 2.1 provides some good news with regard to HIV/AIDS, malaria, and tuberculosis, all of which declined significantly from 2000 to 2012. In terms of treatment, Ugandan health agencies report the absence of a wide range of services and facilities that they would wish to provide (Schmid et al 2008: 1280): higher-level specialist services; diagnostic equipment (such as scans, ultrasound); better laboratories; cancer treatment, as well as ear, nose, throat, dental, and eye care; improved services to rural areas (especially with respect to ambulance services and deliveries); and more antiretroviral treatment and prevention of mother-to-child transmission. A moment's reflection on the preceding list reveals how basic some of these gaps are in terms of treatment. All of this relates back to the general poverty that persists mainly in rural areas, relatively low educational levels, and government underperformance mostly in the health sector.

What, then, can be said of the combination of state, society, and health care in Uganda? An unfortunate causal pathway involving state and society is quite easy to draw here: lack of adequate health care/poverty → ill health → low productivity → poverty/lack of adequate health care (Natala 2006: 139). Central elements along the pathway include "high rates of HIV and AIDS, slow private-sector development, ongoing political instability in the north, heavy reliance on international aid and weak institutional and human capacity" (Schmid et al 2008: 126). In the specific case of Uganda, the regional political instability is due to the impacts of the rebel group called the Lord's Resistance Army and ongoing and violent civil conflicts in neighboring South Sudan and the DRC. Thus, limited economic means combine with health challenges in a self-reinforcing vicious circle.[8] As a key part of that story, consider specific factors that limit access to health facilities (Natala 2006: 145): the lack of drugs in health facilities; the inadequacy of medical personnel; inadequate health sector funding (see also Schmid et al 2008: 127); and the relationship between environmental sanitation and the incidence of diseases. These shortcomings combine to limit the provision of health care and reflect problems that begin with government ineffectiveness and widespread poverty, and ultimately pervade society.

Public health in Uganda is defined by its national Health Sector Strategic Plan as "the science and practice of protecting and improving the health education, control of commutable diseases, application of sanitary measures and monitoring of environment of hazards" (Natala 2006: 143). The first Health Sector Strategic Plan came into being in 2000 and, like its successors, the specifics covered the following five years. The Health Sector Strategic Plan definition encompasses the multiple and interlocking dimensions of health care. Its concept formation includes both mental and physical elements—witness the incorporation of education as well as sanitation. Moreover, this comprehensive definition of public health also encompasses prevention, control, and management, along with treatment.[9] The Ministry of Health, according to Plan III, "takes a leading role and responsibility in the delivery of curative, preventive, promotive, palliative and rehabilitative services to the people of Uganda"; provision of services is "decentralized with districts and health sub-districts (HSDs) playing a key role in the delivery and management of health services" (Ministry of Health, Government of Uganda 2010: 2). In sum, the Ministry of Health defines health in a way that shows awareness of the concept's multifaceted nature—even if action does not always live up to intention.

Given limitations on services provided by the state, it is essential to examine other ways in which Ugandans access health care. Among non-governmental possibilities in society, the religious sector quickly

---

[8] One critical ingredient about access, which tends to be overlooked in the academic and policy-related literature, is distance to a health-care facility. This particular challenge became more salient during the interview process in each state included in the present study.

[9] The development of Health Sector Strategic Plan III, the most recent incarnation (2010–2015), reflected a range of concerns, such as issues of international health, newly emerging diseases, and climate change. Plan III also notes that the MDGs played a role in moving forward (Ministry of Health, Government of Uganda 2010: 1).

comes to the forefront. Around the world, aside from a few exceptions among the developed states, the trend is upward with respect to religiosity (see, as described in Chapter 1, the findings of Norris and Inglehart [2004]). A major cause of this religious resurgence is the fact that secular ideologies in so many developing states have failed upon implementation (Toft et al 2011: 13). Uganda is not an exception. As noted already, the limited capacity of state facilities leads citizens to seek health care from non-state sources. The president cut the Ministry of Health budget by 13.5% in 2012/2013 in order to pay the military—a clear message about what is viewed as most fundamental from a political standpoint. Other signs, however, point in a more favorable direction regarding government efforts to carry through on Health Plan III. For example, in September 2015, the Parliament of Uganda and the Inter-Parliamentary Union signed a memorandum of understanding that emphasizes "matters affecting the health of women and children coming top on its agenda." Activities to be accomplished include: "a background paper on maternal, newborn and child health; drafting and tabling legislation; raising awareness among citizens on issues of maternal, new born and child health, among others" (*New Vision: Uganda's Leading Daily* 2015). The story goes back and forth regarding the government—mixed signals are the norm regarding a commitment to health care.

Uganda is typical of Africa in the centrality of religion to everyday life. The majority of Ugandans are Christian. The distribution of adherents is 84% Christian (Catholics 40%; Anglicans 37%; others 7%) and 12% Muslims, with attendance at religious services estimated to be almost 80% (World Trade Press n.d.: 11; see also Schmid et al 2008: 126). Table 3.5 details religious statistics for the three countries in this study. Religion also tends to be quite syncretistic—combinations of belief systems are commonly encountered—and "indigenous African traditions survive as a compelling force in the society" (World Trade Press n.d.: 7, 11; see also Asante and Mazama 2009). For example, the Lugbara ethnic group believes that the dead may send sickness to remind the living that they are "acting custodians for the Lugbara lineages and their shrines" (Asante and Mazama 2009). In a more general sense, traditions are "grounded in the relationship of the living with ancestors," with the Luo ethnicity as a prime example in that sense (Asante and Mazama 2009). "Most African communities," as Orach (no date) observes, "rally more easily around religious organizations than government." Thus, religious organizations could play a critical role in addressing the health-care needs of Uganda's population.

Unfortunately, religion in society also creates the potential for harm. Consider, respectively, the collective and individual levels. Uganda fell prey to regional, religiously framed strife that left a legacy of violence. The Lord's Resistance Army, a violent social movement led by the self-styled religious figure Joseph Kony, inflicted savage violence on Ugandan society in a struggle against the government that spanned decades. Kony claimed to speak for God and created a political theology with elements of Christianity and Acholi (ie ethnic) nationalism (Sandal and Fox 2013: 14, 136). The Lord's Resistance Army "fused politics and religion" and drew on a mixture of religious beliefs to validate its actions (Chatlani 2006/2007: 281). For example, the Lord's Resistance Army claimed "to make its warriors 'bulletproof' by the use of incantations and charms" (World Trade Press n.d.: 17). The words of one observer reflect the virtually unanimous reaction from Ugandans and international observers alike: "the LRA [Lord's Resistance Army] has brutalized the nation" (Chatlani 2006/2007: 298). Gulu in the central north is just emerging from two decades of civil war; over 90% of the region's population became displaced, with 1.5 million ending up in refugee camps (Schmid et al 2008: 133). The Lord's Resistance Army's long campaign of violence finally ended but not without great loss of life and other costs.[10]

For the individual person, religion might seem to have a curvilinear relationship with public health. Religious observance can divert attention from personal problems as people "think of the good they can do for others" (Kagimu et al 2013). Thus, in Uganda, religious groups are prominent in health care and are an important means of messaging. When carried to an extreme, however, religious beliefs and activities can be harmful to a person's mental and physical health (Kagimu et al 2013). A positive effect exists up to a point, after which the relationship involving religiosity and health issues reverses and becomes negative. Fanatical devotees to a religion may be deceived by false health promises or, in the most extreme of cases, become followers of violent social movements.

Uganda's context, to sum up, intertwines weak government performance in providing services with long-standing poverty. These two traits reinforce each other and impact upon health; pernicious effects then reverberate throughout the state and society. It becomes interesting to look at how civil society groups—notably, those of the

---

[10]   Haynes (2013: 302), however, lists Uganda among several likely African targets for transnational Islamist militancy, which does not bode well for the future.

religious variety—might play a role in health care. This process starts with a look at the academic literature so far.

Religion and health care in Uganda: what we know so far

Mental and physical health, essential concerns at both the level of the individual and society as a whole, reveal connections to religion. "Religiosity," as Kagimu et al (2013) assert, "is one of the psychosocial determinants of health." Religion in Africa is "integral to people's lives and religious entities are deeply involved in the health sector" (Schmid et al 2008). The religious element in health care emerges as a priority for further study and Uganda is no exception.

Orach (no date) provides an overview of religion and health care in Uganda back to1897, the year Anglicans founded the first health facility. The study observes that it is "not known precisely how many traditional medicine practitioners and spiritual healers are operational" (Orach no date). More should be learned about: (1) the connection of religion with the practice of modern medicine; and (2) the role of traditional, religiously oriented healing.

While limited in quantity, the studies that can be identified suggest an important role for religion in relation to health care. The expansion of religious-based facilities "seems to have been stimulated and accelerated in response to certain situations in Uganda"—a "vacuum created by the decline in public health care service and by political instability" (Orach no date). This process reflects the lack of both quantity and quality at the state level regarding health care. A recent estimate places the faith-based health sector in Uganda at about 30% of facilities, with the majority belonging to Catholic and Protestant churches (Boulenger et al 2012: 66). The "PNFPs [private not-for-profits] have been part of the Sector Wide Approach (SWAp) arrangement since 1999" (Orach no date). Religious facilities are regarded as significantly more trustworthy than those in the public sector (Orach no date); for example, Schmid et al (2008: 133) report that nurses trained at PNFPs are regarded as better than those educated through the Ministry of Education. In addition, within marginalized rural areas that lack government services, contributions from the faith-based sector are especially notable (Boulenger et al 2012: 68).

Limited provision of functional resources and ongoing corruption in government has led to persistent unmet needs and some degree of response in terms of the faith-based provision of health services. PNFPs, in a word, are essential. Health services provided by these agencies are predominantly community-based, primary and secondary health services, though some include tertiary hospitals. Many of the agencies reported serving large numbers of outpatients monthly (ie over 10,000 outpatients, with some having as many as 17,000 outpatients), though others were much smaller in scale, serving 60 outpatients a month. Over two thirds offered dispensary services and these provide for a range of between 100 and 20,000 patients per month. While a few of the facilities provided inpatient care to fewer than 100 patients a month, several are much larger in scale, with between 500 and 3,000 patients on a monthly basis.

To acknowledge the negative side of things as well, however, patrons of PNFPs are required to pay significant fees, so the expense is greater than at public facilities. PNFPs do try to limit costs to the extent possible, with one approach being the use of volunteers (Schmid et al 2008: 141–143).

Government cooperation with PNFPs is evident in the public health sector of Uganda. As Tolchinsky (2013) observes, "the Ugandan Government has heavily incorporated certain FBOs [Faith-Based Organizations] into the national health delivery system, through several public–private partnership programs." The PNFPs contribute to "policy and systems-related dialogue and formulations" (Orach no date). From a government standpoint, such activity helps to fill important gaps; politically speaking, Faith-Based Organizations may even be stabilizing in terms of public perceptions and the degree of satisfaction with the order in place. This is because, as mentioned earlier, these organizations include civil society, provide a needed health service, and are often perceived as less corrupt than government clinics.

Public and private sector connections for health are well established. The Inter-Religious Council of Uganda is a network that brings together five different denominations. Founded in 2001, the Inter-Religious Council of Uganda facilitates inter-denominational dialogue on issues of common interest and has five core institutional members: the Catholic Church in Uganda; the Uganda Muslim Supreme Council; the Church of Uganda (Anglican); the Uganda Orthodox Church; and the Seventh Day Adventist Church Uganda Union. Consultation through the Ugandan Catholic Medical Bureau, Ugandan Protestant Medical Bureau, Ugandan Muslim Medical Bureau, and Ugandan Orthodox Medical Bureau is important to the government–religious partnership at an operational level. More than 75% of PNFPs belong to one of the first three preceding religious umbrella bodies—Catholic, Protestant, and Muslim—that have been part of SWAp since its outset (Orach no date). The United Catholic Medical Bureau and United Protestant Medical Bureau are more than

50 years old and connect faith-based efforts with the national public health system. These entities "are well managed and have a strong influence in governmental health policy" (Orach no date). About 37% of the PNFP health facilities are affiliated with the Ugandan Christian Medical Bureau and 31% with the Uganda Protestant Medical Bureau; 7% of the PNFP sector is managed by the Ugandan Muslim Medical Bureau, and the recently created Ugandan Orthodox Medical Bureau holds a small share (Orach no date).

These medical bureaux perform a wide range of essential health functions. The bureaux facilitate health units in a general way and offer technical support on the management of human and other resources. They also engage in raising and distributing funds. The United Protestant Medical Bureau and United Muslim Medical Bureau co-manage a small sub-grant program and the United Catholic Medical Bureau has provided extensive analysis on the costing of services. These are just examples of what the bureaux have accomplished (Schmid et al 2008: 130) and strengthening existing partnerships is therefore a strategy with much to recommend it (Orach no date).

Limitations are also apparent with regard to cooperation between the private religious and public health sectors. Consider the results from field research that focused on two faith-based hospitals involved in contracting agreements with recipients of the US President's Emergency Plan for AIDS Relief (PEPFAR) (Boulenger et al 2012: 66). While the contracts played a positive role in an overall sense, respondents at the hospitals also saw drawbacks, notably, with regard to a lack of "adaptation to the national context," a dearth of connection with national structures, failure to learn from past experiences, and the lack of transparency to others (including the Ministry of Health) (Boulenger et al 2012: 67, 69).

What about traditional healing as the other part of the story regarding health care and religion? It is estimated that traditional healers provide primary health services to about 60% of the population—an important role (Schmid et al 2008: 128). Approximately 145,000 traditional healers—more than the 90,000 workers formally employed in the biomedical sectors—are active in Uganda. They are "respected in their communities" and regarded as potentially health-effective and affordable alternatives to more conventional medicine, but "official recognition and more widespread collaboration" on the part of public providers is still lacking (Schmid et al 2008: 129, 130). The result may be that the whole is less than the sum of its parts.

Traditional and modern health practitioners have formed an organization, Traditional and Modern Health Practitioners Together against AIDS (THETA), to coordinate efforts against AIDS. There are some signs of collaboration emerging between the conventional health sector and traditional birth attendants, for example, in the district of Mukono. An obstacle to teamwork with traditional birth attendants, however, is that referral of a patient to a health center causes loss of income and possibly even the market as a whole (Schmid et al 2008: 129, 136, 137). The institutionalization of traditional practices within the overall health system is at an embryonic stage.

Discussion of religion and health care has so far focused primarily on the institutional level (with modest attention to traditional healers), at which some positive, highly practical traits emerge. Faith-Based Organizations seem to be coordinating efforts with each other and the government through medical bureaux. Coordination with traditional medicine could be improved but some degree of organization already exists even here. What, in turn, can be said of mechanisms connecting religion with health outcomes?

Results from a major project on religiosity and health prove to be enlightening about religiosity and health-oriented behavior. Based at Makerere University in the capital city of Kampala, a research team of medical professionals has produced consistent and highly informative results through survey research regarding the connection of religiosity with HIV/AIDS (Kagimu et al 2011, 2012a, 2012b, 2012c, 2012d, 2013). These studies have focused on Muslims (Kagimu et al 2012b, 2013) and Christians (2012a) individually and in comparison with each other (Kagimu et al 2011, 2012c). The bottom line is important: *religiosity is associated with lower rates of HIV.* While it is beyond the scope of this review to describe each study in detail, the most central aspects of research design deserve closer attention because of both the significance of the results and what they suggest regarding causal mechanisms at the individual level.

Survey research by the Makerere team focused on young people in the Wakiso District in Central Uganda, an area surrounding the capital city and adjacent to Lake Victoria. For example, Kagimu et al (2012a: 19) relied on a sample collected from July to December 2010 that included 4,268 youths from 15 to 24 years of age. The research team interviewed and tested these participants for HIV infection and took a random sample, for purposes of comparison, which included 106 with infection and 424 as controls. Table 3.2 enumerates the dimensions of religiosity on which the Makerere research team focused in respective studies. Subjects responded to 33 questions about religiosity that included spirituality, practices, coping, commitment, and various other aspects (note also religion-specific queries for Christians [question 30] and Muslims [questions 31–33], respectively).[11] Thus, the Makerere-based investigation of religiosity is comprehensive and also tailored to the Ugandan context regarding the most common religious affiliations.

Results from the respective Makerere-based studies convey a preference and positive role for religiosity. Logistic regression analysis shows HIV infection as negatively connected to the following behavior and traits: prayer, one sexual partner, and both parents being alive (Kagimu 2012a: 23). In a study focusing on Islamic youth, the Sujda—prostration during daily prayers (see Table 3.2, item 31)—served as "the main objective parameter of religiosity measured in the study" and revealed a close connection with safe behavior such as abstaining from sex, being faithful in marriage, and eschewing alcohol and narcotic drugs. (It should be noted that the Sujda is taken as a sign of credible commitment to the practice and also the tenets of Islam; the presence of the mark *itself* is not taken to be the causal agent.) The risk of HIV for those without Sujda was about three times as high as for those with the mark on the forehead due to the head touching the ground during prayer (Kagimu et al 2012b: 283, 287; see also Kagimu et al 2013). In another study, HIV infections revealed a high frequency "among respondents who were not circumcised, did not abstain from sex, had multiple sex partners, etc." (Kagimu et al 2011: 709).

Kagimu et al (2012a: 22–23) report that higher levels of religiosity, measured in the following ways, are associated with significantly lower HIV infection rates:

- daily spiritual experiences (asking for God's help in daily activities; feeling guided by God in daily activities; feeling thankful for God's blessings);
- private religious practices (praying privately other than at church);
- religious commitment (trying hard to be patient in dealings with oneself or others; trying hard to love God with all of one's heart, soul, and mind);
- organizational religiosity (frequency of church attendance); and
- overall self-ranking (extent that one considers oneself religious).

---

[11] Measurement for each item, as per this example, is as follows: "I feel guided by God in the midst of daily activities": 1 (many times per day); 2 (every day); 3 (most days); 4 (some days); 5 (once in a while); and 6 (never or almost never). In all instances, category 1 (what could be termed highly religiously observant) is compared to 2–6 in combination (less religiously observant).

Table 3.2: Religiosity dimensions measured among Muslim and Christian groups

Daily spiritual experiences	1. I feel God's presence. 2. I find strength and comfort in my religion. 3. I desire to be closer to God. 4. I feel God's love for me, directly or through others. 5. I ask for God's help in the midst of daily activities. 6. I feel guided by God in the midst of daily activities. 7. I feel thankful to God for my blessings.
Private religious practices	8. How often do you pray privately in places other than a church or mosque? 9. How often do you watch or listen to religious programs on TV or radio? 10. How often do you read the Bible/Qur'an or other religious literature? 11. Do you read the Bible/Qur'an in the language you understand? 12. How often do you fast according to your religious denomination? 13. In your lifetime, how many times have you performed pilgrimage according to your religious denomination? 14. How often do you give charity to the needy according to your religious denomination?
Religious coping	15. To what extent is your religion involved in your understanding or dealing with stressful situations?
Religious commitment	16. I try hard to keep all my promises and agreements with others at home, work, and during leisure in accordance with my religious teachings. 17. I try hard to avoid telling lies to others in all my conversations at home, work, and during leisure in accordance with my religious teachings. 18. I try hard to be trustworthy in all my dealings with others in life at home, work, and during leisure in accordance with my religious teachings. 19. I try hard to be humble in all my dealings with others in life at home, work, and during leisure in accordance with my religious teachings. 20. I try hard to be patient in all my dealings with others and with myself at home, work, and during leisure in accordance with my religious teachings. 21. I try hard in my life to love my Lord God with all my heart, with all my soul, and with all my mind in accordance with my religious teachings. 22. I try hard to immediately apologize if I wrong someone. 23. I try hard to implement my religious teachings in all my life at home, work, and during leisure. 24. I try hard in my life to love my neighbor as I love myself in accordance with my religious teachings.
Religious beliefs/values	25. I believe in God and his angels. 26. In my religion, sex outside of marriage is prohibited.
Organizational religiosity	27. How often do you go for religious services at a church/mosque? 28. Besides religious services, how often do you take part in other activities at your place of worship?
Self-assessment of religiosity	29. To what extent do you consider yourself a religious person?
For Christians only	30. Wearing a cross.
For Muslims only	31. Has Sujda (the hyper-pigmented spot on the forehead due to prostration during regular prayers). 32. Wearing a Muslim cap (males only). 33. Wearing the long dress called Hijab (females only).

Source: Kagimu et al (2012d: 289).

This list invites a discussion of causal mechanisms at the level of the individual. Socio-demographic drivers of HIV are identified as youth, never having attended school, being out of school, and loss of one or both parents, while behavioral factors include sexual activity, multiple sexual partners, not using condoms in sex outside marriage, sex during menstruation, drinking alcohol, and using narcotic drugs for recreation (Kagimu et al 2012a: 23). These factors combine to create a disposition toward risk-taking behavior and acting upon it.

Religion can serve to counteract such forces. Religious beliefs—in the present context referring to Islam—can set "definite standards of right and wrong as a way for people to identify acceptable guidelines for behaviors" and provide "motivation for adhering to the standards" (Kagimu et al 2012a: 24). Also, as religious teaching that promotes self-control is available in all world religions (Kagimu et al 2012b: 289), the results here possess general relevance.

Table 3.3 displays what Kagimu (2012) labels as the "ABCDE of HIV Prevention." The individual-level items combine safe practices with a basis in religion (items A, B, and D), science (C), and both (E). Note that HIV infection is less prevalent among Muslims compared to Christians as conveyed by survey results (Kagimu et al 2012b: 287). The likely interpretation of that difference concerns consumption of alcohol and subsequent risk-taking. Muslims become less likely to contract sexually transmitted diseases as a result of the basic lifestyle decision regarding the non-consumption of alcohol. A 2009 Pew Research Center survey nonetheless revealed that a clear majority (61%) of Ugandan Christians viewed drinking alcohol as morally wrong (Pew Research Center 2010: 272, question 85).

Now consider the level of policy regarding religion and the promotion of public health. Inter-religious cooperation "increases social capital that can be used to reduce HIV transmission in accordance" (Kagimu et al 2011: 709). The workshops held by the Islamic Medical Association of Uganda provide an excellent example. These workshops on safe health practices include Christian community educators as well as the Islamic Medical Association of Uganda sponsors. "The Imams and their assistants," as Kagimu et al (2012b: 283) point out, had been "trained to use a curriculum with both scientific information and Islamic teachings, in the process of educating their communities." A wider range of participants beyond Muslims could participate and receive health benefits through greater awareness of safe practices disseminated to society.

Additional research supports the position that the involvement of religious organizations is important to a health project's survival and

Table 3.3: ABCDE of HIV prevention

Category	Content
A	Abstaining from sex before marriage and abstaining from sex outside marriage, in accordance with God's guidance.
B	Being mutually faithful in a monogamous marriage or being mutually faithful in a polygamous marriage, in accordance with God's guidance.
C	Condom use in appropriate circumstances, in accordance with God's guidance.
D	Diini (religiosity) in the home, at work, and during leisure, especially regular prayers and fasting, in accordance with God's guidance.
E	Educating and encouraging: (1) the promotion of a combination of HIV prevention using behavioral, biomedical, and structural means; (2) patience and perseverance in adherence to ABCDE; and (3) partnership with all stakeholders, in accordance with God's guidance.

Source: Kagimu (2012).

sustainability in many places (Muhirwe 2012: 142). Faith-Inspired Institutions in Uganda provide a wide range of youth-friendly services that, in turn, are associated with greater usage of health treatment services. Youth corners at health facilities, to cite one example, contribute to reducing reluctance among young people to seek assistance (Muhirwe 2012: 138).

Based on the results obtained by Kagimu et al (2012a: 24) and related studies, one policy implication seems straightforward: an approach that "involves education of communities using scientific knowledge supported by religious teachings" pays off. Consider Table 3.4, which conveys the "five pillars" approach to HIV/AIDS prevention from the Islamic Medical Association of Uganda. Once again a combination of scientific (item 2) and religious (items 1, 3–5) components is clear to see. The policy implications of this profile are discussed more completely in Chapter 6.

Consider some further possibilities identified by a health expert, one of the interviewees for this book. Religion can provide a support system that facilitates good health. Forums and roundtables that bring together policymakers with leaders from the religious and medical sectors could therefore be valuable in promoting health-care access and even outcomes.

Summing up what is known so far begins with the observation that religion matters significantly with regard to health care in Uganda. At the national and regional levels, PNFPs are essential and significantly coordinated with government efforts toward health care. Traditional, religiously oriented healing is important but somewhat apart from the rest of the health-care system. Religion also impacts significantly on health at the individual level. The influence is largely positive, but fervent political beliefs impair judgment and promote authoritarian, "black and white" thinking. People with the most intense religious beliefs may be more prone to deception or the use of less efficacious providers of health care (eg witch doctors), as well as joining violent

Table 3.4: Five Pillars of the Islamic Approach to HIV/AIDS from IMAU

Everyone should remember the five pillars of how to use religiosity (Diini) for HIV prevention which are supported by the new scientific information. These pillars are the things everyone should remember and do to prevent new HIV infections on a regular basis. They should be at the tips of the fingers of everyone.

Pillar	Content
1	Pillar 1: Believe in, trust and obey God, and His messengers. This pillar is supported by the new scientific data, showing that people with higher levels of the following dimensions of religiosity related to God have lower HIV infection rates compared to those with lower levels of these dimensions. 1. Ask for God's help amidst daily activities 2. Feel guided by God amidst daily activities 3. Feel thankful for God's blessings 4. Try hard to love God with all one's heart, soul and mind.
2	Learn and use scientific knowledge, information and wisdom about HIV/AIDS prevention in accordance with God's guidance. This pillar is supported by scientific data showing that people with higher levels of religiosity have lower HIV infection rates when compared to those with lower levels of religiosity.
3	Learn and use faith teachings and practices that support HIV prevention in accordance with God's guidance. This pillar is supported by scientific data showing that people who pray several times daily have lower HIV infection rates compared to those who do not. For Muslims this pillar is supported by scientific data showing that people who pray several times daily, resulting in getting Sujda, have lower HIV infection rates compared to those who do not.
4	Participate in partnerships for HIV prevention by listening to and using good advice from parents, religious leaders, health care workers and community leaders in accordance with God's guidance. This pillar is supported by scientific data showing that people who listen to or watch religious programs on radio and TV usually given by religious leaders, are more likely to have good behaviors that are expected to reduce new HIV infections compared to those who do not. It is also supported by scientific data showing that youth who have both parents alive and presumably giving good advice to their children, have lower HIV infection rates when compared with the youth who have lost one or both parents.

5	Use the concept of self-control for HIV prevention according to God's guidance and resist Satan that brings temptations by regularly asking and praying for God's help. For the Muslims, use the concept of self-control (Jihad Nafs) for HIV prevention according to Allah's guidance and resist Shaitan that brings temptations by regularly praying for Allah's help and seeking refuge in Allah. This pillar is supported by the scientific data showing that people who frequently try hard to be patient and exercise self-control in their dealing with themselves and others at home, work and during leisure in accordance with God's guidance, have lower HIV infection rates compared to those who have lower levels of this behavior. In addition, people who fast as a means of self-control in accordance with their faith teachings have lower HIV infection rates compared to those who do not. For the Muslims, people who fast the month of Ramadan or more as one of the means of self-control, in accordance with their Islamic faith teachings, have lower HIV infection rates compared to those who do not. People who frequently pray also had lower HIV infection rates. For the Christians, these people are more likely to pray in accordance with the teaching of Jesus Christ and include asking for God's protection from Satan as follows: "Do not bring us to hard testing, but keep us safe from the Evil One" (Holy Bible, Matthew, Chapter 6, verse 13). For the Muslims, these people are more likely to pray in accordance with the teachings in the Glorious Qur'an including asking for Allah's protection from "Shaitan" (Satan) whenever confronted with temptations reciting: *"If a suggestion from Shaitan assails your mind, seek refuge with Allah; for He hears and knows all things. Those who fear Allah, when a thought of evil from Shaitan assaults them, bring Allah to remembrance when lo! They see alright"* (Holy Qur'an, Chapter 7, verses 200–201).

Source: Kagimu et al (2012b: 282).

social movements.[12] It is important to note that positive health–care outcomes are associated with the use of modern medicine with an underlying religious motivation and world view.

Faith-based health provision and behavior: preliminary findings from interviews

General importance of religion

Religious belief has an important impact on both health–care provision and health-seeking behavior. Although a few interviewees criticized religion's role in health care, not one person objected to the idea that faith mattered for both provision and consumption. Interviewees at Makerere University's School of Public Health, for example, quickly

---

[12] The term "witch doctor" is controversial and some may be offended by its appearance. Within the pages of this study, however, references to witch doctors follow on from interview material and academic literature. In other words, the term is not introduced independently, but instead exists within ongoing dialogues about health care in Africa.

Table 3.5: Christian population as percentages of total population

Country	Ethiopia	Mozambique	Uganda
Percentage of 2010 population that is Catholic	0.7	28.4	42.2
Percentage of 2010 population that is Protestant	19.2	27.1	44.4
Percentage of 2010 population that is Orthodox	43.5	—	—
Percentage of 2010 population that is Christian	63.4	56.1	86.7
Percentage of 2010 population that is animist	2.2	29.4	2.3
Percentage of 2010 population that is Muslim	34.6	18	11.5

Sources: Pew Research Center (2011) and Brown and James (2015).

confirmed Uganda as a religious state and drew attention to its Christian heritage of spiritual and medical care. They further observed that, at the individual level, religion plays an important role and may account for health decisions in perhaps half of the population.

Religion and health provision

Uganda's history provides an important context in which to understand the nature of religious belief and health care. Prior to the 1900s and the advent of British rule, as described by an employee at the United States Agency for International Development (USAID) all health care followed traditional means, primarily using herbal medicine. During the British Protectorate of Uganda (1894–1962), European missionaries arrived, leading to the rapid growth of the Christian faith among Ugandans. The missionaries also built schools and hospitals. From the 1870s onward, the colonial government and missionaries introduced Western medicine. Thus, there is a long tradition of health care for Ugandans that is faith-based *and* Western in nature. Even in the independence era, Ugandan churches have remained, according to the USAID employee, "in a key position when we talk about health care." This is because of their high status and the fact that Faith-Based Organization health centers reach deeper into rural areas and the quality is claimed to be higher than at government facilities. The USAID employee estimates that, currently, something like 45–57% of national health-care needs (involving modern medicine) are met by faith-based facilities and mainly by Catholics and Anglicans, who offer a range of services.

One faculty member of the School of Public Health at Makerere University estimates that 40% of health facilities in the country are faith-based, primarily hospitals. These facilities provide about 70% of training for health professionals. As a former employee at a Catholic hospital, the professor spoke to the higher quality of care at such facilities, with specific reference to a "sense of discipline" and lower likelihood of theft. Officially, government hospitals are free—but the professor claimed that under-the-counter charges exist.

Based at a rural Catholic hospital to the south-west of Kampala, one doctor asserts that "PNFPs are helping government to offer the services. The government even seconds some staff to Nkozi [Hospital]." For such reasons, observes a health consultant, PNFPs create the potential for greater professionalism and continuity in the health sector.

According to an employee with a health centre, Village Health Teams play a valuable role as a bridge between the government and community regarding health provision. It is a national policy that all villages have a Village Health Team. The Village Health Team links health institutions, notably, including faith healers, to each other and the people. Members of the Village Health Team are selected by the people of a village; they are volunteers but have some training from medical professionals. Team members spontaneously visit anyone known to be sick in order to counsel them. Village Health Teams are valuable in fighting myths, such as the persistent belief that ultrasound can be harmful to the child or mother. In a more general sense, a health consultant sees potential in Village Health Teams for improvement in management, leadership, and organization at the local level. In turn, if these possibilities work out, liaison with the national government could also be improved.

Village Health Teams entered into the discussion at another health centre as well. The question of interactions with traditional healers came to the fore. This type of medicine produced a negative response whenever mentioned; traditional healers are "harmful and expensive." The centre thus favors a scientific approach; from the quite secular point of view found there, in all likelihood, personal reasons best explain why people go to traditional healers at all.

Consultation with available reports would suggest a mixed view of Village Health Teams. A summary from the Uganda Village Project (2015) points out that by 2009, Village Health Teams still did not exist, for instance, in the Iganga District, north-east of Kampala and near the Kenyan border. As a result of limitations in government services, the

Uganda Village Project intervenes at the community level to meet the need for Village Health Teams (Uganda Village Project 2015). A report from the Ministry of Health in March 2015 tells a more detailed story about Village Health Teams, with the glass half full or empty, perhaps, depending on the point of view. On the one hand, it is estimated that a total of 179,175 Ugandans are Village Health Team members. With World Vision as one example, 109 implementing partners are now active in Uganda (Ministry of Health, Government of Uganda 2015: 5, 6). On the other hand, 30% of Village Health Team members do not have basic training, the strategy is unevenly implemented across districts, and activities are hampered by a lack of funds (Ministry of Health, Government of Uganda 2015: 5, 7).

A government official asserts that the government is *trying* to provide services. The government has budgeted for health care, albeit at a level compromised by greater allocations to the military, but *implementation* is weak. Regrettably, corruption plays a harmful role. The government official observes that "civil servants are the problem" and more monitoring is needed with regard to the provision of services. The president, according to the minister, continues to put pressure on Members of Parliament (MPs) to stay in touch with public needs at the ground level. A health consultant reinforces that point by citing sustained participation by MPs as a key to success in bridging the gap between national and local levels with respect to health-care provision.

Traditional methods for the provision of health care are also very important in Uganda. Ugandans make important distinctions, however, between the types and motivations of those providing such services. These categories include traditional herbalists, witchcraft, and traditional birth attendants. Traditional religion, it should be noted, gradually became associated with the negatives of witchcraft and child sacrifice. Therefore, witchcraft is illegal in Uganda under the colonial-era Witchcraft Act 1957. Crimes such as child sacrifice are also addressed under other laws. Access to health education at a more uniform level throughout the country, according to a health consultant, is the most promising path away from the most pernicious activities associated with witchcraft.

An employee from a Muslim hospital in Kampala identifies three different types of faith healers. Those of the first type, spiritual healers, do not support people attending health facilities because they believe in witchcraft. People who visit spiritual healers are often mismanaged until "the condition gets out of hand" and then people might visit a health facility. This is not acceptable in Islam. Second are herbalists, some of whom, according to the employee at the Muslim hospital, do good work. This is acceptable in Islam as long as it is not accompanied by any "funny conditions" that have spiritual connotations. Traditional birth attendants comprise the third type. Many women deliver with them at home and then attend health facilities for child immunization. These observations add up to a balanced view of traditional healing, with the first point drawing attention to danger and the second and third points acknowledging more positive effects.

A district health officer estimates that about 30% of people attend churches and use traditional healers—even 5–10% of MPs. The officer notes that there are many miracle healing churches, such as the Miracle Centre Cathedral. The Cathedral teaches that God intervenes for spiritual healing, but it is not completely opposed to conventional medical treatments.

The district health officer further distinguishes spiritual and traditional healers from each other. Spiritual healers hold traditional African beliefs and use herbs, rites, and sacrifices. Traditional healers incorporate the religious and spiritual component into their healing but not rites. There is no formal credentialing for faith healers; success is what matters in attracting patients. From the government's point of view, this is a service to be valued because it fills a gap—put simply, who would care for these people otherwise?

The district health officer also explained that an umbrella organization exists for traditional healers and birth attendants that is situated under the community and gender department. The officer differentiated two types of traditional healer: herbalists and those who use "different means." The latter seemed implicitly to mean those who use religious rites or even sacrifices as part of their treatment regime. While the government asks traditional healers to register, the district health officer observed that many do not and the authorities are thus unable to work with them. The district health team requests that traditional healers refer certain cases, such as tuberculosis patients, for immediate treatment. The officer noted that it is difficult to remove traditional healers from even the cases most obviously beyond their purview, so the adopted strategy is to "be their friend."

An employee from the Ministry of Health refers to traditional medicine, based on traditional African religion, as "indigenous." The Ministry of Health employee sees a shift away from traditional approaches. Quacks *do* exist, but the problem with witch doctors is fortunately dissipating. Medications provided by traditional healers are generally herbal and made from locally available fruits and the like. Such medications have shown success in reducing malaria rates, but the role of the herbal approach remains uncertain for the future. The vast range of herbs in use is not fully understood, across the board, by those prescribing them. It is already known that indigenous herbs and synthetic drugs tend to help with different problems. A 2005 article by the Makerere Medical School, for example, examined the use of medicinal plants by traditional healers to treat male sexual impotence and erectile dysfunction. The study documented 33 plants used for treatment. Two particular plants, *Citropsis articulata* and *Cola acuminata*, are the most frequently prescribed. The study also noted that "70–80 percent of the Ugandan population still rely on traditional healers for day-to-day health care" (Kamatenesi-Mugisha and Oryem-Origa 2005). It is fair to say that the breakpoint between Western and herbal medicines is not always clear. The study advocated the creation of some type of board to administer pharmacopeia resulting from local medications.

According to the Ministry of Health employee, an export market already exists in the West for herbal remedies. Some treatments for cancers are being tested and there is a need to "industrialize" to produce remedies for the local market and beyond. Uganda imports 99% of modern drugs used, so trying to replace these with locally available treatments would have great value.

Through a translator, the midwife in a village within a very poor, rural area in Central Uganda answered a series of questions about her work and the role of traditional healing in general. (Translation went back and forth between English and Swahili.) If mothers in the village need help, they are more likely to visit her than anyone else. Most mothers do go to the hospital now to give birth, but the midwife still does one or two deliveries per month. She reports that her sole formal training occurred in a hospital back in 1979. The midwife also claims to send complicated cases directly to the hospital. Some women consult traditional healers before trying to see her, but she only assists those who come to her *first*. If they have gone to a traditional healer initially, she sends them to the hospital. The midwife reports, along those lines, that traditional healers try to provide her type of service.

Unique in the process of interviews, time with a "traditional healer"—also a herbalist—pointed toward the hybrid nature of such practitioners. Elements of science combine with traditional Ugandan medical customs to sum up the experience. The healer's lavish homes and polygamous lifestyle suggested a lucrative profession. He had been designated for his role by family at the age of seven and had risen to become district representative for the national organization of traditional healers. The drugs he used himself included alcohol, tobacco, and unspecified contents of one of many bags that contained herbs.

His summary of treatment through herbs made sense by intuition, on average, given experience with their effects. (The traditional healer grew some of his products on about two acres of land.) He claims to recognize maladies that require hospital assistance and *does* consult with Western-style doctors. Problems that, from his point of view, are neither spiritual nor treatable with traditional medicines are referred to the local hospital.

Religion and health-seeking behavior

An MP for Ndorwa West, Kabale District, expresses uncertainty about how people's belief in miracles might affect their pursuit of health-seeking behavior. Pentecostals, for instance, firmly believe in miracles; some have faith in a divine ability to cure illness directly, whereas others see this as action by God as manifested through doctors. Pentecostalism, according to the MP, is expanding most rapidly among all churches in Uganda because its adherents target young people (ie those under 35) by using technology and "modern ways": singing, dancing, and emphasizing the role of Christianity in the contemporary world. The MP sees this as having an impact on other religions, with Catholicism and other faiths having to adapt to this competition.

According to the district health officer mentioned earlier, most people's first point of call for health services is a herbalist. Only if this does not improve their condition will they then go to a health center. At first, the district health officer suggested that this might be due to the relative proximity of traditional healers. However, the officer then acknowledged that such choices do not just occur in rural areas; rather, the preference is acted upon everywhere and seems culturally embedded.

The district health officer notes that patients make health-seeking decisions based on money. While government hospitals are free, there are frequently "stock-outs," which means that it becomes necessary to buy drugs from private pharmacies. PNFPs charge but are generally better supplied. The officer also observes that there is a culture of self-medication, with patients simply going to pharmacies without visiting a health facility.

The previously noted professor also believes that choice of facility is based on financial considerations and the privileges associated with where one works. Another Ugandan professor focuses on modern as well as traditional medicine and confirms that point through personal experience in deciding upon services to obtain when recently welcoming a child into the family. In sum, choices are about services, comfort, and affordability; those who can will go to a private facility.

Doctors at the Ministry of Health acknowledge the significant role of religious beliefs in health-seeking behavior. Muslims particularly use herbalism, though some associate that type of medicine with witchcraft. Religious leaders exist on both sides of this issue. No database exists for herbalists, however, and one of the doctors just noted argues that the government needs to have a *registry* that shows "who is doing what." A health consultant, in fact, identifies a lack of information in an overall sense as one of the greatest challenges to public health, especially in impoverished rural areas.

An administrator at a Muslim hospital further observes that religious leaders are important and highly respected, and their "words weigh a lot." Most Muslims are sufficiently informed to go about daily life, according to the administrator, but it is the responsibility of religious leaders to provide deeper interpretation on issues such as health to guide the community; this requires impressive knowledge of science *and* Islam. The mosque is a valuable venue for disseminating health-related messages: "It is done and important." Muslim NGOs can also help with this. At a higher level, the hospital administrator confirms that efforts are coordinated at the Inter-Religious Council of Uganda.

A health consultant extends the point regarding the Inter-Religious Council of Uganda into a call for greater recognition of, and action upon, the essential *interdependence* between health-care efforts in the governmental and religious sectors. To some degree, each sector operates on its own, which, in turn, produces results that might have been better with more coordination. Thus, an entity such as the Inter-Religious Council emerges as a point of contact that the Ugandan government might emphasize as it considers the future deployment of resources.

Traditional and spiritual healing

Negative attitudes over witchcraft are widespread. According to an MP, African traditional religion is dying off. Witchcraft still exists, but witch doctors and those patronizing them are a shrinking minority. The MP reports that people from their constituency are overwhelmingly Christian or Muslim.

Sources at a university, however, put forward a different view about the continuing viability of religious alternatives to modern medicine. Traditional religion is often combined with Christianity and impacts upon beliefs and actions about health. For example, there is even belief in the value of child sacrifice, which is believed to occur most often in the Central region of the country. Church leaders complain about parishioners following traditional beliefs as well. So-called "double agents" are numerous. People look for miracles, especially if what they are hearing in a formal church setting does not resonate with them. According to the team at the School of Public Health, this may prompt the dissatisfied party to consider witchcraft. A health consultant adds, in this context, the observation that a more structured approach— emphasizing classes and public forums—could help to deter people from resorting to practices that have no scientific basis and could prove harmful to health outcomes.

Traditional religion, according to a professor, is pervaded with fraud because it lacks official recognition. The professor draws a contrast with its recognized place, for example, in Benin. Little documentation exists regarding who is animist or about traditional religious practices in general. Such approaches are undervalued and looked down upon. However, some people with HIV use traditional medicine, so religion plays a problematic role there. This is connected to the overall question of access to Western medicine. Outside of Botswana, for instance, is it reasonable to guess that the average African can get the medicines they need?

A doctor (and health administrator at the sub-district level) claimed that people do not visit a traditional healer for contraception because they have "failed in that area" (ie pregnancies ensue despite would-be spiritual efforts at prevention). However, traditional healers are visited for other conditions, such as infertility. Traditional healers often charge more than the hospital: 40,000 Ugandan shillings (or about USD11) for a traditional birth attendant versus 35,000 Ugandan shillings (or slightly less than USD10) for an institutional delivery. Women's families often pressure them to attend a traditional birth attendant. Most people attribute infertility to spiritual reasons and this is also true for other conditions that show no physical manifestation.

The doctor just described also reported, with some amusement, that witch doctors also attend the hospital. Some witch doctors are strictly spiritual, while others are herb-oriented and still others are both. Only very educated and committed Catholics do not attend traditional healers. The doctor only learned that modern conception ran contrary to Catholic doctrine when attending a university that belonged to a Catholic group. The doctor had also been asked questions about their faith by university friends that he could not answer, so he took advantage of available training to learn more.

Expressed by an employee of Health Centre IV, located in a rural area south-west of Kampala, is an altogether negative view of traditional healers. Put simply, they are associated with "collateral damage." The employee reported, quite emphatically, *no* contact between clinics and traditionalists; the interviewee claimed that any information moving back and forth had been transmitted through patients. When asked about traditional healers, employees at Health Centre III responded even more negatively: they laughed openly. The centre employees acknowledged that a "few" patients seek traditional medicine and reported that, in particular, the clinic offers counseling to persuade pregnant women from going down that path. They added that Village Health Teams do not influence the conduct of traditional faith healers. Instead, communication is with community members.

A political figure—who was decidedly more critical of faith-based health-care provision—observes that faith-based facilities are profit-seeking. Ultrasound, for example, is a service for which mothers must *pay* in faith-based clinics. While religious facilities are higher in quality, they are relatively expensive. The politician finishes up on this point with a rhetorical question: what are Faith-Based Organizations doing for the *poor*?

Evaluation of the role of religion in health care

A doctor sees important benefits from church attendance: socialization, support groups, and employment contacts. A political figure concurs regarding the positive impact of religion on health, for example, lower levels of stress. The politician frames sin as harmful activities and diseases such as alcoholism, promiscuity, and HIV. This interviewee connects faithfulness in marriage with religious belief, which thereby serves as a preventive measure regarding sexually transmitted diseases.

A doctor reports that, based on results from a cross-sectional study, regular church attendance is associated with reduced alcohol consumption. This is important because alcohol consumption is "very high" in Uganda; the generalization is true mainly among men and increases with age.

A professor put forward some positive points regarding the impact of religion on health. Discipline and respect inculcated in an individual can help to promote a healthier lifestyle. A principal instance would be the role of religion in discouraging youth from the risk-taking behavior associated with nightlife. This helps with personal productivity and, in turn, facilitates entry into society as one of its positively contributing, respected members.

An employee from the government's Department of Disease Control and Environmental Health reinforces that argument. Religion can be a voice for health campaigns, with avoidance of sexual relationships outside of marriage and abstinence as mutually agreeable messages. Religious leaders, who are held in high esteem, can join forces with parliamentarians and university leaders to represent the needs of their people; hospital construction would be just one instance of a significant priority.

An employee from the government Ministry of Health notes that religious leaders can play an important role in mobilizing people and disseminating health messages. There is a general perception that religious facilities provide better care than those of the government. (Interestingly enough, religious health facilities started off in the most disadvantaged locations, beyond the reach of government, and the poorest people still rely on faith-based health services through clinics and hospitals.) The government provides support to the faith-based services. Religious entities are also represented in the government's health policy planning advisory committee, which constitutes a public–private partnership.

The health delivery economics differ for traditional health care in comparison to Christian or Muslim health-care facilities. Traditional birth attendants, according to a district health officer, are asked to refer all pregnant women for institutional delivery. However, doing this constitutes losing their livelihood, so it does not happen very often.

A doctor from the Ministry of Health, like others, sees herbalists as sensible regarding their limitations—but witch doctors are not. The doctor asserts that church leaders are respected and thus provide a good avenue for the dissemination of medically sound advice. An example is provided from South-Western Uganda: a bedridden man with malaria and HIV. People prayed over him and someone told the doctor about the man's illness. The doctor and other leaders talked to the man; they accepted his faith but also told him that he needed to go to the hospital.

Health professionals at Makerere University's School of Public Health see religion's negative role manifested in behavior such as the non-acceptance of blood transfusions, which leads to high mortality. Prayer in lieu of medication is "injurious to health." Along similar lines, an employee from USAID sees "a huge danger and vulnerability on the part of people who seek health care from traditional healers." This is because it takes so much effort to convince these practitioners that they cannot manage a particular condition and really need to release the client to a doctor. As a result, patients may die because a disease becomes too advanced by the time they obtain conventional medical care. The employee from USAID provided a personal example of the danger posed by such behavior. This matter concerned the daughter of a colleague's sister. The family had prayed for her to get better; when she finally visited a health facility, her CD4 count[13] had reached nine cells/mm³.

Religion can also play a role at the level of public policy, sometimes with indirect effects that are significant and potentially harmful to health. Consider a Bill opposed to homosexuality, supported strongly by a politician among the interviewees. The political figure endorsed the legislation, entitled the Uganda Anti-Homosexuality Act, on the basis of belief that homosexuality is a sin and sees the Bill as designed to accomplish four things:

- to stop the promotion of homosexuality;
- to stop the recruitment of children into homosexuality;
- to stop the funding of homosexuality; and
- to ensure that any future international commitments with relevance to homosexuality are debated in Parliament.

It almost goes without saying that the preceding list of priorities would be controversial in developed states. The Parliament of Uganda passed the Bill in December 2013 and President Musevini signed it into law on February 24, 2014. The Act, however, had a short lifetime; on August 1, 2014, the Constitutional Court of Uganda ruled it invalid. During that process, the Act—and evangelicals involved with supporting it—received considerable media attention, which resulted in verbal attacks and rebukes from Western governments and even threats to end financial aid.

Should aid be provided to Uganda when its legislature passes such anti-gay measures? This is not the time and place to answer that question. Indeed, one interviewee regarded the query from a moment ago as one-sided. The other side of the question, from the interviewee's point of view, would concern whether Ugandans, many of whom do not accept homosexuality as a part of their culture, should be expected to liberalize on that issue in order to receive foreign assistance. Looking at both sides of the issue could be more informative in identifying the best set of policies for Uganda as a whole.

---

[13] CD4 T-cells are white blood cells that fight infections such as those caused by bacteria and viruses.

Processes and outcomes

Processes

Religion matters in Uganda, and health care is no exception. The story is mixed but not without positive elements and hope for the future.

With regard to the provision of health care, the role of religious entities is crucial in light of a tepid performance by government. Some degree of integration is emerging at both national and local levels with respect to religious and secular, government-based, health care. At the national level: the Inter-Religious Council of Uganda, THETA, and several bureaux exist; Village Health Teams are playing a positive role at the local level; and there is significant liaison with PNFPs. While the whole continues to be less than the sum of its parts, coordinated efforts are underway and a foundation exists for further improvement. The essential interdependence of the religious and governmental sectors in health care needs to be acknowledged more directly in order to facilitate progress.

Health-seeking behavior is influenced strongly by religious beliefs. An overwhelming example is the role played by herbalists as a "front line of defense" in the war on illness. Many Ugandans consult herbalists and make use of religious facilities that provide modern medical treatment. These actions reflect the sustained importance of local effects on health-seeking behavior.

Traditional and spiritual healing are significant components of health care in Uganda. Herbalists and traditional birth attendants play a key role in filling gaps created by limited government services. While witchcraft exists and is denounced as quite harmful, it may be on the wane.

Evaluation of the role played by religion in health care is difficult in an overall sense because both positive and negative stories can be told. Regarding the favorable side, many Ugandans receive treatment from religious health centers and hospitals that compares favorably to what can be obtained from government facilities. Moreover, the limited nature of government provision makes the resources from the religious sector absolutely vital. Also positive is the role played by many herbalists and spiritual healers, and it certainly helps when religious views cause adherents to eschew risk-taking behaviors that could damage their health.

Unfortunately, religion can also play a harmful role with regard to health care. Those with extreme religious views may engage in acts of violence against either the government or other citizens who are seen as enemies for doctrinal reasons. Intense devotion to particular kinds of religious beliefs could also cause someone to refuse treatment from modern medicine when it is essential to their recovery from one malady or another. Witch doctors, who provide services with no scientific basis and even engage in human sacrifice, still exist.

Overall, it might be said that the glass is more than half full regarding religion's role in the process of health care for Uganda. This is a significant overall message from both the academic literature and interviews. Perhaps memory of the Lord's Resistance Army will cause a national aversion to violent social movements that claim a religious basis. Coordination of efforts from government and religious entities is underway in the health sector. Many religious individuals also abstain from practices that cause health problems. In sum, today, Uganda is a state and society with the opportunity to build in a positive way on what has been accomplished so far with respect to the religious contribution to the health system.

Regarding the frame of reference provided by the Social Determinants of Health, it is clear that the point of intuition about religion is right on target. Health-related processes are impacted upon across the board by religion. Demand exceeds supply for health care as supplied by the government and, in a quite rational way, Ugandans turn to the faith-based sector. Religious entities provide life-sustaining support and there is no sign of their role diminishing with time.

Outcomes

Given this study's concern with country-specific progress and outcomes with regard to MDGs 2 and 4–6 (regarding the gender-equal attainment of primary and secondary school education) and MDGs 5 and 6 (women's reproductive rights and the provision of HIV treatments), it is appropriate to focus on Uganda's progress on these measures. The review looks initially at national developments and shifts to a gender-oriented approach to detect important nuances behind the aggregate figures.

With respect to MDGs 2 and 3, consider specifically gender equality regarding enrollment in, and graduation from, primary and secondary education. The "good news" is that each sex showed an enrollment rate of more than 80% in primary school. That figure has declined from 2002 when the measurements began, where male and female enrollment had been right around the 85% mark (Uganda Ministry of Finance, Development and Economic Planning 2013: 18). However, the on-time completion rate for both remains in the single digits. The adult literacy rate of those aged 15–24 as of 2010 stood at 77% for men and 75% for women, a large improvement over the course of the decade (Uganda Ministry of Finance, Development and Economic Planning 2013: 18). As of 2012, the share of girls to boys in primary education reached 100%, but only 85% and 79% for secondary and tertiary education, respectively (Uganda Ministry of Finance, Development and Economic Planning 2013: 20).

With respect to the legal status of reproductive rights, the situation in Uganda is quite murky. The only permissible grounds for terminating a pregnancy are if the life or health (physical or mental) of the mother are endangered (Center for Reproductive Rights 2011). The current situation is summed up effectively by a report from the Guttmacher Institute (2013a): the unsafe termination of pregnancy is uncommon, with varying levels of risk. Interpretations of the law are ambiguous and medical providers can therefore be reluctant to perform an abortion.[14] A more recent piece by Berer (2017) shows that Uganda's Constitution and Penal Code conflict with each other on abortion. While Uganda claims to have a national policy on abortion, "it is not supported in law and is not being implemented" (Berer 2017: 17). Published in 2015, the Standards and Guidelines on the Prevention of Unsafe Abortion specified boundaries for legal abortion in Uganda; the policy was withdrawn the next year, attesting to executive power in African politics (Berer 2017: 17–18).

Assessments by the UNDP, Planned Parenthood, and Guttmacher Institute, among others, convey a strong sense that women in Uganda live between the "official" reality of access to contraception/abortion and their own problems of access. Thus, we may say that Uganda's women unofficially cannot access the official framework, rendering official statements moot. A Guttmacher Institute (2013b) report confirms that observation:

> One estimate of abortion incidence in Uganda comes from a 2003 study that reported an annual abortion rate of 54 abortions per 1,000 women of reproductive age, or one abortion for every 19 such women. This rate is far higher

---

[14] The Ugandan Constitution states that "abortion is permitted if the procedure is authorized by law," with the 2006 National Policy Guidelines and Service Standards for Sexual and Reproductive Health and Rights asserting that "pregnancy termination is permissible in cases of fetal anomaly, rape and incest, or if the woman has HIV." These conditions, in practice, prove difficult to implement without some degree of confusion and therefore aversion among medical personnel.

than the average rate for Eastern Africa (36 abortions per 1,000 women). Most providers have to work in clandestine environments. (Singh et al 2005)

A UN study revealed the maternal death rate to be 1,200 per 100,000; unsafe abortion is listed as the second leading cause of maternal mortality (at 35%) in 1986 (UN 1986). Jagwe-Wadda et al (2006: 9) showed that about 15 of every 1,000 women of reproductive age received treatment for complications from induced abortions in Ugandan health facilities each year.

The Guttmacher Institute (2015) observed that "an estimated 45% of all women experiencing complications from abortion do not receive care at a facility" and the proportion is even higher for those under the poverty line. Lack of post-procedure care obviously results in a high mortality rate (Guttmacher Institute 2015). In 2005, Singh et al noted that "about 525 of every 1,000 women would require treatment for complications from an induced abortion during their 35-year reproductive lifetime." (Singh et al 2005: 187).

The authors of MDGs 5a and 5b, the Maputo Protocol, and the Beijing Platform on Women's Rights, among others, recognize an ironclad link between a mother's ability to access reproductive care (while pregnant and at other times) and the health of her pregnancies and their outcomes. It is therefore impossible to speak of MDGs 5a and 5b in isolation from each other, as the international women's health movement recognized when it pressed for the addition of MDG 5b in 2005.

Regrettably, more than half of pregnancies in Uganda are unintended, with nearly a third of them ending in termination. Women report having families of at least two more children than desired (while they prefer an average family size of four, the average size is six). This figure is termed "excess fertility" by family planning specialists and Uganda has one of the highest rates in sub-Saharan Africa.

With a high rate of "excess fertility," unplanned pregnancies, and deaths from abortions, Uganda reveals the need for a better, more evenly distributed, network of reproductive health services across the country. Studies by the Guttmacher Institute show that while contraceptive use among married women doubled between 2000 and 2011, that figure rose from only 14% to 26% (Guttmacher Institute 2013a). Use of modern contraceptive methods in Uganda obviously remains too low to address needs for the effective spacing and prevention of births. The rates of contraception do not come even remotely close to the goal of at least 75% prevalence typically found in the Global North (UN

2015b). The Guttmacher Institute also reported in 2011 that one in three married women had an unmet need for contraception. Overall, the UN's Department of Social and Economic Affairs (UN 2015b) report shows most of Africa at the highest rate of unmet contraceptive need (24%), as opposed to a global average of one half that figure.

Just as it is impossible to separate good outcomes for women either experiencing pregnancy or during the rest of their lives from access to good care, including contraception, it is very difficult to separate MDG 5 from the effects of MDGs 2 and 4. UNICEF shows that women with lower rates of education, especially in Africa, experience: (1) higher rates of unintended pregnancy and all of its complications (ie maternal and neonatal deaths and injury); and (2) lower access to contraception than their more educated counterparts (UNICEF no date; Guttmacher Institute 2015). UNICEF confirms that access to education and good maternal nutrition results in a much-reduced death rate for their children under five. One bright note is that the teenage birth rate has declined from 204 per 1,000 teenagers (ie between 15 and 19) in 1995 to 135 in 2011 (Uganda Ministry of Finance, Development and Economic Planning 2013: 26).

The Guttmacher Institute also mentions the trend for women to go to traditional practitioners. At least one district in Uganda has outlawed traditional birth attendants on the basis of high death rates for women (Kabayambi 2013). It appears that women are badly served by traditional practitioners such as birth attendants. Unfortunately, the vast majority of sub-Saharan African states are not on track to meet their goal in MDG 5a of having a majority of births attended by skilled personnel (UNICEF no date). On the one hand, the rate of skilled birth attendants went up from 38% to 58% between 1995 and 2011. On the other hand, the maternal death ratio per 100,000 was only reduced from 507 to 438 (Uganda Ministry of Finance, Development and Economic Planning 2013: 24). The Uganda MDGs report also shows that, in the early 21st century, among 553 hospitals surveyed, only 3% who supposedly offered emergency obstetric care could do so. The reasons for maternal death are hemorrhage (at 42%) and obstructed/prolonged labor (at 22%)—both of which suggest lack of timely access to skilled personnel (Uganda Ministry of Finance, Development and Economic Planning 2013: 25). With respect to MDG 6, it turns out that 45% of HIV-infected mothers in sub-Saharan Africa transmit the infection to their children (UNICEF no date).

While the Uganda report claims progress on reversing incidences of malaria and tuberculosis since the early 21st century, the spread of HIV/AIDS has not declined along all dimensions. Among males and females aged 15–24, females are typically three times as likely to report being HIV positive than males. Unfortunately, women are also much less likely to report using a condom during their "last risky sexual encounter" by at least 10% (Uganda Ministry of Finance, Development and Economic Planning 2013: 27). One bright note in this area is that while a large gap existed between males and females when it comes to understanding the links between risky sex and the HIV infection, it had disappeared by 2011. However, the figures are still below 40% of respondents for each sex (Uganda Ministry of Finance, Development and Economic Planning 2013: 27). Finally, the report shows that while the MDG had been that 80% of the population should have access to anti-retroviral drugs, the percentage was 62 in 2012, which the Ugandan government claimed was "on track" (Uganda Ministry of Finance, Development and Economic Planning 2013: 27).

Significant change in the numbers just reported seems unlikely in the near term without a major cultural shift regarding the position of women in Ugandan society, most notably, in relation to their maternal role. Government policies, moreover, sometimes make the provision of maternal health more difficult because valuable services that reside outside the mainstream may be ruled out of bounds.

Information on outcomes is more limited than processes, so assessments must be tentative. At the very least, however, it is clear from Guttmacher Institute assessments that women do not have universal access to the strong, value-free prenatal and comprehensive reproductive care envisioned by MDGs 5a and 5b. Traditional, untrained midwives, unsafe abortions, and lack of contraception all contribute to the figures of higher-than-desired family size mentioned by women.

Since fertility is high relative to Western rates, the position of women is affected quite significantly by policies and beliefs related to reproductive health. It is disturbing that an interviewee, a member of a Village Health Team, reported the persistence of a myth that ultrasound can be harmful to the mother or child. Shortages of institutional support intersect with the persistence of traditional birth attendants to create a problem for women's health. While traditional birth attendants are asked by district health officers to refer women to a hospital for delivery, to do so challenges their livelihood and is thus not the norm. Moreover, traditional healers, according to an interviewee in a good position to know, try to provide services that include delivery but are not qualified (ie at least at the level of a midwife) to take such actions. On the provision side, it is reported that faith-based clinics charge expectant mothers for ultrasound. This creates obvious disadvantages for those who are not well off in obtaining the best available care.

While overall movement on the MDGs is positive for Uganda, not all is well. Several problems have been identified regarding reproductive rights for women. In addition, Sigsworth and Kumalo (2016) have pointed out that the 2003 Maputo Protocol, the African Union's Protocol to the African Charter on Human and Peoples' Rights on the Rights of Women in Africa, has suffered from patchy implementation. This is perhaps not a surprising record given limited resources and the contestation over multi-level frameworks in general. As Sigsworth and Kumalo (2016: 4) note, the Maputo Protocol states clearly the important equation of ensuring gender equality, which, in turn, affects women's social, economic, and political empowerment, and thus their human security in all forms.

For example, one part of the Maputo Protocol explicitly calls for an end to female genital mutilation. Uganda passed a law prohibiting the practice in 2010, giving 10 years' prison time to anyone practicing it and seven for anyone abetting it (Mutebi 2016). Yet, there are still remote groups, mainly associated with the Sebei or Sabiny ethnic groups of Sudan and Uganda, who practice female genital mutilation. The Sabiny are part of the Kalenjin people. It is believed that 50% of the Sabiny and 95% of the Pokot people, living in the mountainous and forested areas of Eastern Uganda (including the Kapchorwa district), still practice it (Masinde 2013).

Ugandan state strategies to combat female genital mutilation, as Mutebi reported for the *Daily Monitor*, have focused on reaching out to Sabiny elders who practice it. These elders, in turn, become included in development projects as a way to compensate for their lost income. Thus, Uganda is one of the African countries on the forefront of making a reality of at least the anti-female genital mutilation part of the Maputo Protocol.

Overall, according to the Mid-Term Report on the African Women's Decade, there are still areas of concern for maternal, women's, and children's health in Uganda. One chief problem is that women and children have been disproportionately affected by the periods of internal conflict, and form the majority of displaced persons (Make Every Woman Count 2016: 81–84). Related to the violence and disruption, "many Ugandan women will face rape, domestic violence and early and forced marriage in their lifetime." (Make Every Woman Count 2016). While the Ugandan Parliament passed a 2010 Act against family violence, as of 2016, the laws had not yet been implemented effectively (Make Every Woman Count 2016: 81–84).

Unfortunately, Uganda remains one of the countries with the highest rates of HIV infection (and AIDS), which is thought to be related to the high percentage of forced, youthful marriage and internal displacement through conflict. The role of the Ugandan military should also be noted because of its very high prevalence of HIV and role in spreading the virus within and beyond the state's borders. Moreover, infection rates have been rising. Female genital mutilation, of course, also contributes to propensity to sexually transmitted diseases and HIV due to genital tearing and scarring. With one of the highest rates of adolescent marriage globally, it is encouraging that Uganda has been able to lower its overall fertility rate and teenage fertility rate. Another fortunate outcome of health-care resourcing is that, as of 2016, 58% of women were attended by skilled attendants during the birthing process (Make Every Woman Count 2016: 81–84). Another positive trend is that Uganda passed its "first ever National Strategy to end Child Marriage and Teenage Pregnancy," developed with NGOs and UN consultation, which "aims to create a society free from child marriage and teenage pregnancy" (Make Every Woman Count 2016).

Summary

Religion is central to the story of health care in Uganda, in terms of both provision and health-seeking behavior. Ugandans view health in a holistic way. Traditional and spiritual healing exist alongside Western-style medicine and can combine to produce positive results. Awareness exists among the latter type of health providers that coordination can be beneficial to patients. While witchcraft still causes health problems in Uganda, it is on the decline by all accounts. Large-scale violence in the name of religion had also occurred, but the Lord's Resistance Army is a thing of the past and no similar movement seems on the horizon.

With regard to outcomes, progress is evident regarding the MDGs. Shortcomings, however, are apparent when the overall figures are viewed in terms of women's health. On balance, Uganda is improving on health care, and religion is a largely positive part of that story.

4

Mozambique

Overview

This chapter turns its attention to religion and health care in Mozambique. The two basic questions from Chapter 1 will be answered, at least in part, by the research reported here: (1) "How does religion factor into the Social Determinants of Health?"; and (2) "What is its connection to outcomes?"

Before moving ahead to answer those questions systematically, it seems appropriate to foreshadow the basic contributions of the chapter. Mozambique, an especially poor state, had a Marxist government that suppressed religion for decades. People retained their religion, however, and it influences health care quite significantly in contemporary Mozambique. Health planning from the government exists but is challenged by persistent poverty and underdevelopment. Christian and Muslim Faith–Based Organizations play an important role in fighting HIV/AIDS and the provision of health care in general. Pentecostalism is rising and plays a controversial role in its engagement with modern medicine. People still seek traditional health care and even combine such visits with more Western-style treatments from health centers and hospitals. Women's health is somewhat better than in some other African states—one of the few positive legacies from the previous Marxist regime. In sum, religion turns out to be essential to both the provision and consumption of health care in Mozambique.

The Republic of Mozambique gained independence from Portuguese colonial rule in 1975. Due to a lack of Portuguese capital or commitment to develop its colony, Mozambique ended up less economically developed at the time of decolonization than other countries in Africa. A decade-long struggle for independence aggravated the lagging economy of Mozambique. Its level of economic development was also impacted by disastrous political and economic policies adopted by the new Marxist government, as well as a 15–year civil war that commenced soon after independence. In 1994, the civil war ended and the country initiated political and economic reforms that have led to tangible socio-economic improvements. Nonetheless, Mozambique remains among the world's poorest countries.

According to United Nations (UN) data, in 2009, 60.7% of the population lived on less than USD1.25 per day (calculated in terms of purchasing power parity). The impact of economic growth and development following the end of the war is evident. In 1996, the year for which the first figures after the end of the civil war are available, 80.6% of the population lived on less than USD1.25 per day. By 2002, this figure had dropped to 74.7%. Furthermore, wealth in the country is unevenly distributed. In 2008, the World Bank estimated that Mozambique had a Gini coefficient[1] of 45.6, compared to an average of 43 in sub-Saharan Africa.

Primary research reported in this chapter took place largely but not entirely in Maputo, the capital city of Mozambique, in June 2011.[2] Those interviewed included academics, government officials, and individuals with non-governmental organizations (NGOs). Their positions and dates for the interviews are located in the Appendix (see p 196). Due to the particular circumstances of Mozambique's history and political trajectory, research material on the impact of religion regarding the provision and supply of public health is sparse.

Interviews with government and civil society individuals have produced valuable insights about religion and health in Mozambique. Implemented solely in Maputo, a pilot quantitative assessment yielded interesting results that are explored in this chapter. The survey instrument designed to elicit information on religious belief and health-seeking behaviors is also included. The survey was not employed in Ethiopia and Uganda due to practical difficulties encountered in the Mozambique pilot project.

This chapter continues in four additional sections. The chapter's first section offers a broad overview of the Mozambican context. The second section provides a brief summary of existing research on religion and health care in the country. The third section presents interview material on the role of religion in public health processes in five subsections: (1) the general importance of religion; (2) religion and health provision; (3) religion and health-seeking behavior; (4) traditional and spiritual healing; and (5) an evaluation of the role of religion in health care. An additional subsection surveys outcomes on

---

[1] The Gini coefficient is a measurement of income inequality in a country.
[2] Robert Lloyd conducted primary research in Mozambique. He has 25 years of experience with the country as head of a non-governmental organization (NGO), speaks Portuguese, and has had numerous articles on the politics of the country published. He also lived in Maputo for two years.

the basis of the Millennium Development Goals (MDGs). The fourth and final section proffers conclusions.

Context

Mozambique is a "Y-shaped" country located largely in the tropics along the south-eastern coast of the African continent facing the Indian Ocean. The shape reflects Portuguese colonial-era control of the coastal area and inland settlement along the Zambezi river valley. The gap in the top of the Y is filled by the independent state of Malawi, formerly a British colony. Mozambique is bordered on its north by Tanzania, Malawi, and Zambia, and along its western frontier by Zimbabwe, South Africa, and Swaziland. As of 2014, the country's population stood at approximately 25 million people contained in 799,380 square kilometers—about twice the size of the US state of California. The largest city and political capital is Maputo, located in the far south of the country and along the coast. The economic capital, and second city, of the country is Beira—a port city farther to the north.

Mozambique is a poor country, even by African standards. Most Mozambicans reside in rural areas working as farmers on small plots of land. Half of the population is below the poverty level. Its per capita income is USD1,200 (purchasing power parity). However, in the past decade, the country has enjoyed strong economic growth of approximately 7% per year, fostered by earlier economic reforms and fueled by subsequent foreign direct investment in so-called mega-projects such as the Mozal aluminum smelter and Temane and Pande gas fields (CIA World Factbook 2016).[3]

What is now Mozambique took gradual form during the colonial era that began in the 1500s. The coastal areas fell under Portuguese control as that European state pioneered trade routes around Africa to Asia. In the first half of the 20th century, Portuguese increasingly settled in Mozambique. Large numbers of Mozambican men also provided labor for the gold mines in neighboring South Africa. Mozambique became independent in 1975 after a decade-long struggle against Portuguese colonial rule. At independence, the country contained a sizeable European population who had been occupying most positions in government and entrepreneurial roles, virtually all of whom left the

---

[3] This increased level of performance might represent regression to the mean, at least to an extent, given the severe losses to the economy from prolonged civil war and the resumption of pre-war agricultural activity.

colony at that time, crippling the country's economy. According to Egerö (1987), by 1975:

> an estimated half of the Portuguese community had left the country, carrying with them all that could be taken away and destroying the rest. They were to be followed by most of the remainder already in the year after Independence, leaving the new government with an economy extremely dependent on an increasingly hostile neighbour, South Africa, and with only the rudiments of a functioning bureaucracy.[4]

The source of revenue from Mozambican gold miners working in South Africa also dried up.

The new Marxist-led Frelimo government then implemented collectivist policies that further weakened what little had been left of the economy. The post-colonial regime also supported liberation movements in neighboring Rhodesia (current-day Zimbabwe) and South Africa. Importantly, this led to reprisals by these countries and their active support for a rebel group—known as the Mozambican National Resistance (Resistência Nacional Moçambicana) or by its Portuguese acronym, "Renamo"—that grew in strength and effectiveness. Renamo engaged in low-intensity conflict tactics specifically targeting Mozambique's economy and provision of social services. The war and a serious drought conspired to bring the country close to collapse by the early 1990s. The widespread and unrecorded laying of landmines in rural areas during the war by government and rebel forces further hindered recovery.

With regard to health in particular, the Marxist government had nationalized medical care, taking over church-run clinics and hospitals and making private facilities illegal. Moreover, anti-government rebels particularly targeted public health facilities as symbols of the Marxist government. As a by-product of the low-intensity conflict from Renamo, much of the health-care infrastructure was destroyed in the war.

---

[4] Consider the construction sector as one example: "decline reflects the wider postindependence economic collapse…. However, the reduced activity was also related to the departure of the settler population and the ensuing collapse in the market in new houses and offices as well as, and most centrally, to legislative changes following independence" (Sidaway and Power 1995: 1471–1472).

A series of World Bank and International Monetary Fund reforms, known as Structural Adjustment Programs, commenced in 1987. These provided desperately needed funds to the country in return for a major restructuring of the economy. In 1990, the government renamed the country from the People's Republic of Mozambique to the Republic of Mozambique, signifying its shift away from a Marxist orientation. A negotiated settlement in 1993 between the government and Renamo formally ended the war, further liberalizing the country politically and economically.

Liberalization of the political system led, for the first time in the country's history, to national elections in 1994. The former Marxist government and the rebel movement (now a contesting political party) basically split the vote, with a slight majority voting for the incumbent party. The results of the vote confirmed an ethno-linguistic split in the country between groups in the north and south. Accounting for 37% of the population, the Makhuwa or Makua–Lomwe is the largest ethnic group (Henriksen 2014: 13). According to Henriksen (2014: 13), the Makhuwa are concentrated mainly "in the northern region of the country, and North of the Zambezi River, particularly in Nampula and Zambezia provinces…. The main group residing south of the Zambezi River is Tsonga, corresponding to about 23% of the total population." As assessed by Manning (2002: 9), polarization of the political arena and dominance by the two former warring parties facilitated a "two-track process of conflict management in post-war Mozambique." The war, according to Manning (2002: 9):

> produced a bipolar division of the political space in Mozambique, which was sustained with remarkably little change during the first post-war decade. There were no significant elite defections from the upper or even middle echelons of either party, and the voter bases of the two parties have remained largely unchanged. Each continued to command overwhelming majorities in its traditional areas of support: Frelimo in the south and far north and Renamo in the five central provinces.

Opposition support for rival presidential candidates gradually diminished in subsequent elections. The most recent national elections took place on October 15, 2014. The ruling Frelimo party candidate, Filipe Nyusi, was elected president with 57.03% of the total votes cast. The opposition Renamo party candidate—and former leader of the Renamo rebel forces—Afonso Dhlakama, garnered 36.61% of the vote. A third-party candidate from the Democratic Movement of Mozambique (known as MDM from the Portuguese acronym for Movimento Democrático de Moçambique) won 6.36% of the total vote. The MDM party broke away from Renamo. Results from the election for the 250-seat Assembly of the Republic appear in Table 4.1, which shows that the opposition parties improved their control of the Assembly of the Republic. While Frelimo retained the presidency, Renamo and MDM are advancing their positions effectively within the legislature. However, Renamo still holds 57.6% of the seats in the legislature.

Today, Mozambique is a *de facto* single-party dominant state with a rapidly growing economy. African states such as Uganda and Ethiopia—the other cases in this study—also fall under that category. Mozambique has been led by Frelimo since independence, as a sole legal party from 1975 to 1990 and as an elected party since 1993. This fits a post-Cold War African pattern, where elections have "resulted in one large majority party, often a second, but quite junior, minority party, and then many fragmented and very small or transitional parties" (Quinn 2016: 167–168).

Mozambique's long period of one-party rule is not unusual in Africa. In Uganda, President Yoweri Museveni's National Resistance Movement has held power since 1986 and the Ethiopian People's Revolutionary Democratic Front has been in office since 1991. South Africa, one of the most democratic countries in Africa, has been under the control of the African National Congress since 1994. The African National Congress has faced no serious political opposition during this time.

Pernicious effects on governance can follow on from one-party dominant rule. For example, Transparency International's Corruption Perception Index for 2013 ranks Mozambique at 119 out of 177

Table 4.1: Election results for 2014

Party	Votes	%	Seats	Seats Gained/Lost
Frelimo	2,575,995	55.93	144	−47
Renamo	1,495,137	32.46	89	+38
MDM	384,538	8.35	17	+9
Other parties	149,812	3.25	0	0
Invalid/blank votes	711,454			
Total	5,316,936	100	250	
Registered	10,964,978	48.49		

countries. It scores the country at 30 out of 100, with zero being corrupt and 100 being clear of corruption (Transparency International 2013).

Mozambique's religious make-up shows similarity to other states in Africa, along with some important differences. The 2007 census provided a general breakdown of religion in Mozambique (CIA World Factbook 2016) and the new compilation from Brown and James (2015) provides more fine-grained data. Given Mozambique's Portuguese colonial history, it is not surprising that approximately 30% of the population professes to be Roman Catholic. A significant percentage (19%) is Protestant, with a number of differing denominations. Evangelical and Charismatic Protestant believers are the fastest-growing group in the country. About 18% of the population is Sunni Muslim, located primarily in the Swahili Coast area of North-Eastern Mozambique. Islam came into the region in the ninth century as Arab traders traded with Africans along the coast, leading to the religion's introduction into that area.

Approximately 29% of the population falls into an "other" category with regard to religion (Brown and James 2015). In an African context, this category is likely made up of individuals who follow African Traditional Religion, with animist as a common designation. Great caution must be used in employing statistics in Africa and these figures should thus be seen as general guides.

What is unique to Mozambique is that although the country may be described as largely Christian, with just over half of the population professing that faith, this figure is relatively low compared to other countries in Southern Africa. Table 4.2 displays the religious percentages by province in Mozambique. This characteristic relates to colonial history, where Christian evangelism—particularly of the Protestant variety—had been suppressed by the Catholic Church. The Catholic Church did not, for its part, evangelize to the same degree as elsewhere in Africa. Moreover, during the Marxist years after independence, religious observance was actively repressed. Given this historical context, traditional African religious beliefs persisted in Mozambique to a degree greater than in other countries.

What about the role of religion in government and society today? The state, in a remarkable policy change from its earlier positions, accepts religious freedom in the country (Lloyd 2011). The 1990 constitution guarantees freedom of religion and places no restrictions on religious observance and education. In recent years, the government has pursued good relations with religious groups while also seeking to separate the two spheres of church and state. Christian and Muslim schools operate

Table 4.2: Religion by province for the population of Mozambique

Religion	Mozambique	Cabo Delgado	Gaza	Inhambane	Manica	Maputo	Nampula	Niassa	Sofala	Tete	Zambezia
Catholic	27.8	36	15.4	24	2.9	16.5	39	26	18.5	21.5	40
Zionist Christian	15.2	0.2	37.5	35.8	4	39.8	1.5	2.6	18.9	17.3	8.6
Protestant	12	1.5	18.8	11.6	3.8	18.2	5.3	7.7	22.4	12.5	11.1
Muslim	17.6	53.8	0.9	1.2	0.2	2.5	37.5	60.9	2.4	0.8	9.7
Total region pop (%)	100	7.8	6	6.2	7	5.8	19.3	5.7	8	8.6	18.7

Note: All statistics are for the year 2007. These figures do not include Maputo City, which is separate from Maputo Province, but has a provincial status as a capital city.

Source: Knoema Regional Statistics of Mozambique.

freely, foreign missionaries receive residency visas, and the government does not interfere in religious organizations' leadership appointments. The government does, however, restrict religious organizations from forming political parties and such parties sponsoring religious groups. The government requires that religious institutions be registered, and the state does not observe any religious holidays as national holidays. During Marxist-rule, Christmas was celebrated as "Day of the Family." Today, the two holidays are celebrated on the same day.

Historical context thus plays an important part in understanding the present role of religion and health care in the country. After independence, the state assumed the dominant role in the delivery of health care, deliberately marginalizing the position of faith-based delivery systems. The relative poverty of Mozambique and the strong role of the state in providing health care have led to close collaboration between the government and foreign donor agencies. For example, writing for Action for Global Health (the German Foundation for World Population), Koenig and Goodwin (2011) evaluate the effectiveness of European Union (EU) development assistance on Mozambique's health sector. They observe that health care in Mozambique has been guided by the government's "Programa Quinquenal do Governo" or Five-Year Development Plan, the most recent of which covered the 2010–2014 period. This plan includes increasing access to health services, especially for rural Mozambicans.

Health policies are contained in a number of government documents. The 2007–2012 Health Sector Plan sets government priorities for Mozambique. Koenig and Goodwin (2011: 8) reported that "cornerstones of the policy are primary health care, equity, and better quality of care." They add, however, that the percentage of government spending consumed by the health sector is not altogether clear. The Ministry of Health estimated the proportion at around 11%. This fell below the Abuja Declaration target of 15%. In 2010, the most recent year for which data are available, 44% of the health sector's budget came from foreign financial assistance. However, external funding such as that from the Global Fund to Fight AIDS, TB and Malaria is also directed to NGOs within the country and not calculated directly into government figures.[5]

The Abuja Declaration[6] was a vow made by African countries in April 2001 to spend at least 15% of their annual budgets on health care. This constituted Africa's direct contribution to meeting the MDGs. The Global Fund is principally a way of pooling bilateral donor aid intended to go towards the treatment and prevention of HIV/AIDS, tuberculosis (TB), and malaria. Pooling the money allows for economies of scale, prevents the duplication of effort, and ensures that expertise is available. While Bill Gates and his foundation had been involved in the initial launch of the Global Fund in 2002, 95% of its money actually comes from bilateral aid agencies in the West. The Global Fund's headquarters are in Geneva.

Figures from the Global Fund to Fight AIDS, TB and Malaria report that, as of 2014, total foreign assistance for Mozambique between 2004 and 2014 had reached USD402 million. Nearly all of the money was

---

[5] https://www.theglobalfund.org/en/
[6] http://www.un.org/ga/aids/pdf/abuja_declaration.pdf

disbursed to combat the two major killers in Mozambique: AIDS and malaria. HIV/AIDS prevalence rates have grown in Mozambique, in part, due to Mozambican migrant laborers that worked in and then returned from South Africa, Zimbabwe, and Swaziland, all three of which have relatively high prevalence rates. The Global Fund has pledged USD690 million. Almost two thirds of that amount (USD445 million) is designated for HIV/AIDS and close to one third has been spent on malaria control. TB (another major disease) and strengthening health systems account for the balance of spending.

Access to health care is an ongoing issue, over and beyond the challenges posed by specific maladies such as HIV and malaria. Koenig and Goodwin (2011) also stated that Mozambique's "Poverty Reduction Strategic Program" reports that "only 36% of people have access to a health facility within 30 minutes of their homes." Furthermore, about 30% of the population are unable to access health services. The Mozambique Poverty Reduction Strategic Program observes that "only 50% have access to an acceptable level of healthcare" (World Health Organization no date). It is not clear from the report, however, what constitutes "acceptable" (Koenig and Goodwin 2011: 23). In addition, "long distances to reach health clinics still affect the poor, especially in rural areas, and the lack of financial means both to cover transportation costs and eventual unofficial fees or bribes to be paid for the delivery services" (Koenig and Goodwin 2011: 23). Finally, Mozambique "also has a severe shortage of trained health professionals. Health sector wage levels have also been a problem with health workers underpaid, and no great incentives provided to locate to more rural locations where unfilled posts remain a problem" (Koenig and Goodwin 2011: 23). This is an ongoing problem throughout Africa and the developing world in general.

Koenig and Goodwin (2011: 25), on a site visit to a rural health hospital near Maputo, report shortages of staff and medicines and a lack of more modern equipment. Medical personnel at the hospital assert that the lack of transport constituted one of the greatest challenges. This impeded the ability of people to access health care because patients also lack sufficient funds to travel to the hospital. The hospital did receive international NGO technical assistance, but it focused on HIV and maternal mortality rather than broader health issues. This was due to the interest of the two international NGOs in this health sector and the hospital's policy of providing free services to pregnant women. It is also noted in the report that Frelimo Members of Parliament (MPs) saw the Abuja goal of spending 15% of the budget on the health sector as "unrealistic and ambitious" (Koenig and Goodwin 2011: 26).

These reports and conditions are reflected in the UN's Human Development Report for Mozambique. The Human Development Index measures a "long and healthy life, access to knowledge, and a decent standard of living" (UN 2013). In 2012, Mozambique's score of 0.327 placed the country in the category of "low human development." The ending of the war in Mozambique and its subsequent economic growth clearly had a positive impact on Mozambique's Human Development Index: the value went up from 0.217 to 0.327 between 1980 and 2012, an increase of 51% (UN 2013). However, the country's standing remains very near the bottom, ranking 185 out of 187 countries and territories.

The World Health Organization reported that Mozambique approved a new Health Sector Plan for 2014–2019. This new plan contains seven strategic objectives.[7] The World Health Organization further reports that the health system in Mozambique is a mix of government, for-profit, and not-for-profit actors. The government provides 60% of the health coverage through state-funded hospitals and clinics in the country. External actors also play an important role in the health-care system. Mozambique has agreements with more than 25 bilateral and multilateral health organizations. To foster better coordination, efficiency, and transparency, the Mozambique government developed a "Sector Wide Approach" to health in 2000. Similar approaches for the health sector have been used in both Uganda and Ethiopia (Brown et al 2001).

Mozambique's context, in sum, presents significant challenges to the operation of an effective health system. Decades of Marxist government produced policies, notably, nationalization, which compounded the problems already posed by poverty. Moreover, years of civil war, with social services and their workers in the crossfire, had clearly taken a toll on the system. In spite of the former Marxist government's efforts to eliminate religion from Mozambique, it persisted into the more tolerant era that exists now. This outcome is fortunate because, as it turns out, the faith-based provision of health care has proven essential to meeting even minimal needs due to limited performance on the

---

[7] The goals are to improve: (1) access to and utilization of health services; (2) the quality of service provision; (3) geographic access between different population groups in accessing and utilizing health services; (4) the efficiency of service provision and resource utilization; (5) partnerships for health; (6) transparency and accountability on the management of public goods; and (7) the health system in an overall sense.

part of government. Mozambique receives ongoing assistance from the international level in combating HIV/AIDS and malaria.

Persistent poverty and underdevelopment, however, remain the greatest challenge to the pursuit of health in Mozambique. These ongoing problems are explained, at least in part, as a legacy of violent civil conflict. Consider the role of land mines in particular:

> Because of the need to protect their land-based interests from the RENAMO insurgency, FRELIMO also used landmines for defensive purposes. In many cases, initial minefields were laid around strategic installations, but often these proved inadequate against attacks. Hence, FRELIMO in many cases continued to add sites until large areas extending well beyond the immediate perimeter of installations were protected. In doing so, they often disrupted a host of land uses. This was particularly devastating to smallholder agricultural land as well as important transportation routes. (Unruh et al 2003: 849)

For such reasons, substantial areas of the best agricultural land in two provinces "have remained uninhabitable or problematic for long periods due to mines" and "as many as 500,000 landmines exist primarily in the most fertile areas" (Unruh et al 2003: 852). Clearly, the presence of landmines bequeathed a harmful legacy.

Religion and health care in Mozambique: what we know so far

For Mozambique, as in many if not most other African countries, information regarding health care and the related effects of religion is sparse. Njihia et al (2012: 10) determine that the degree of religious observance in Mozambique is high compared to a more secular West. Of those surveyed, 83% state religion to be "very important" in their lives; another 15% designate it as "moderately important." Taken together, these data indicate that 98% of Mozambicans consider religion to be important, with obvious implications for the pursuit of health care. Note that the majority (89%) of survey participants are Christian; 5% are Muslim, which under-represents that religion's 18% share of Mozambique's population, and 6% are affiliated with other religious faiths, which also under-represents the 29% figure for animists.

Chand and Patterson (2007) found that Faith-Based Organizations are an important means of effecting significant change with respect to health-seeking behaviors. They cite, as an example, a project in Gaza Province sponsored by World Vision. The organization trained individuals as community health volunteers to function as leaders in "care groups" that comprise 10 people each. Health training includes dehydration, nutrition, immunization, birth spacing, and hygiene. The results of the project showed a significant drop in child mortality due to better and more rapid care and improved nutrition.

Agadjanian (2005) asserts that it is important to differentiate religious denominations in Mozambique—they are not monolithic. His research in Southern Mozambique reveals that Faith-Based Organizations are not homogeneous, but vary between Catholic and Presbyterian "mainline" churches and what he terms "healing" or Pentecostal and Charismatic groups such as the Assembly of God, Zionist, and Apostolic denominations. (Pentecostals make up 11% of the population [Brown and James 2015].) Agadjanian (2005) concludes that members of these churches did, indeed, show some greater awareness of HIV/AIDS messaging and prevention compared to secular counterparts, but this turned out to be even more evident in mainline than healing churches. Agadjanian (2005) suggests that this pattern may be due to social and economic differences between the two groups, with mainline church members having relatively higher socio-economic levels. He also notes some differences in awareness and prevention between male and female members. In general, fluency in Portuguese is higher for males than females.

Research in Southern Mozambique finds that church responses to health challenges such as HIV/AIDS are hindered by capacity constraints. Agadjanian and Sen (2007: 362) argue that policy efforts "to involve religious organizations in provision of HIV/AIDS-related assistance should take into account that organization's resources, institutional goals, and social characteristics." A USAID (United States Agency for International Development) report dated in 2006, however, states that religious involvement had had a *positive* impact on malaria prevention and treatment in Mozambique. The report cited efforts by Anglican Bishop Dinis Sengulane to support a nationwide, ecumenical anti-malaria effort called Programa Inter Religioso Contra a Malaria (PIRCOM), a Portuguese acronym for the Inter Religious Program Against Malaria. The program aimed to train religious leaders in bringing health messaging on malaria prevention and control to a local level. The report stated that PIRCOM was present in six provinces in Mozambique. As a result, 27,000 religious leaders had been trained, enabling them to reach almost two million people in their congregations with important health information.

Religious leaders spearheaded the Inter Religious Program Against Malaria in Mozambique. These leaders believed that they could be effective especially in combating malaria because of their role within the faith community in Mozambican society. This includes the idea that religious leaders are trusted, can foster the widespread mobilization of local communities, and are able to reach into areas of the country where the government has a weaker presence. A proposal from religious leaders to USAID subsequently received funding (WHO 2007).

Efforts of religious leaders have achieved some success in the health sector. According to a USAID follow-up report in 2010, religious leaders assisted in reaching its goals of health messaging, promoting health-seeking behaviors, and bridging religious divisions through a common effort to prevent and control malaria in Mozambique. The effort had been funded by the USAID's President's Initiative in conjunction with the US Centers for Disease Control.

Dube (2009) examines the interaction of religion and health care from a historical perspective. Focusing on the central region of Mozambique, his study argues that colonial-era policies on disease monitoring and health-care delivery to introduce Western medicine had the unintended consequence of encouraging traditional African healing practices. This was due to distrust of the motives of the colonial authorities and their inability to deliver adequate health-care services to meet the needs of people. Thus, Africans remained skeptical of Western approaches to epidemiology and medicine. However, Pfeiffer (2005), in "Commodity Fetichismo, the Holy Spirit, and the Turn to Pentecostal and African Independent Churches in Central Mozambique," argues that more recent community views toward traditional healers in Central Mozambique are not positive. Healers are seen as charging high fees and, at times, having a more malevolent intent toward the individual or other people. These traits, Pfeiffer argues, have led individuals to seek Pentecostal and charismatic churches—perceived as less divisive—for spiritual and physical healing.

With respect to Pentecostalism in particular, Pfeiffer (2011) states that both HIV and Pentecostalism shared similar vectors following the end of Mozambique's civil war in the early 1990s; both moved from neighboring countries into the areas around Mozambique's major cities. Thus, there is a high degree of overlap in beliefs and disease in these geographical areas, and a difference is discernible among Christians of a Pentecostal or Roman Catholic background. Preventive health care, however, is an issue that favors Catholics due to their relatively high presence in health-care delivery and connections with foreign donors. Pfeiffer argues that HIV prevention and treatment efforts have not included Pentecostal churches in these semi-urban areas hit hard by HIV.

Agadjanian (2012: 132) conducted a survey in 2008/2009 that covered all identifiable religious congregations in Chibuto District, with a population of 200,000 and typical among the largely agricultural districts of the Gaza province toward the southern end of Mozambique. The survey included leaders of 678 different congregations. With an estimated rate of 25% for HIV in the province, this malady emerges as a natural point of concern (Agadjanian 2012: 132). The survey reveals that 83% of religious leaders had spoken about HIV/AIDS, primarily about prevention, at least once per month during services (Agadjanian 2012: 133). On the positive side, church messaging helps with mobilizing members for testing and prevention efforts that focus on the avoidance of dangerous objects such as unsterilized syringes, while on the negative side, it is apparent that the problems and challenges of those with HIV are much less discussed (Agadjanian 2012: 135).

Cau et al (2013) present results of their research on how socio-economic status acts as an intermediary variable in assessing the impact of religion on health care. They found a correlation between educational levels and religious belief through examining child survival and health indicators (Cau et al no date). According to Cau et al (2013), belonging to a mainline or Pentecostal church decreases the risk of death for a child compared to the probability regarding non-religious Mozambicans in the Southern Mozambique study. Cau et al (2013) postulate that the difference occurs because mainline churches encourage seeking health care and Pentecostal churches provide a stronger social support network. This social cohesiveness is due to "restricted membership (especially among Apostolic churches), high frequency of attendance and intrusion of religious leaders over members' private lives" (Cau et al 2013: 5). Christian Mozambicans also have higher levels of prenatal visits than their non-religious counterparts (Cau et al 2013).

Academic literature confirms that religion, despite years of facing suppression under the Marxist Frelimo regime, continues to be important in Mozambique. Religious leaders are active in fighting malaria, HIV/AIDS, and child mortality. The next step is to look at evidence from interviews to learn more about how these processes are playing out on the ground.

Faith-based health provision and behavior: preliminary findings

The general importance of religion

Two Mozambican health officials who work on health issues for World Vision noted that, legally, Mozambique is a secular state and thus does not support any religion. These officials affirmed, however, that religious beliefs are very important for Mozambique in understanding health-seeking behavior. Even decades of Marxist rule could not uproot faith from the people of Mozambique.

Officials at the Ministry of Health also affirmed the important of religion and health care. They observed that religious belief influences health. These officials agreed with research presented in an earlier section of this chapter that religious belief also relates strongly to the level of education of the individual. These officials further added that religion is also affected by the regional location of a person. The Ministry of Health officials said that it is important to distinguish among various types of religious faiths in Mozambique in order to understand better the impact of religion on health. Put differently, if you live in the north-east part of Mozambique, you are Muslim. The south is more Christian. Other areas may be more traditional. Traditional beliefs, drawing on pre-colonial African culture, would be more prevalent in the rural areas, but not always. The "cane cities" on the outskirts of the "cement cities" feature lots of traditional adherents. Secularist and modernist beliefs are more restricted to a small number of individuals who live in the large cities and may have had a Western education. By Western standards, at least, almost all of Mozambican society is traditional in that it is largely rural and pre-modern.

These Ministry of Health officials presented two broad categories for Mozambican Christians. The first they termed the "Emerging Churches" (Igrejas Emergentes). These churches practice "miracles" that involve healing. Generally, these are Pentecostal churches that have been heavily influenced by counterparts in Brazil and the US. The officials pointed out one entity as being particularly influential: the Universal Church of the Kingdom of God (Igreja Universal do Reino de Deus [IURD]). The second category the officials termed "traditional." These churches include Presbyterians, Methodists, Anglicans, and Roman Catholics—those that would be called mainline in the US. These churches do not emphasize miracles of healing. The officials thought the educational levels of members of each category to be roughly equivalent, again agreeing with scholarly research. They noted that Muslims on the Indian Ocean coast of the country use both Western-style and traditional healers (*curandeiros*), but do not emphasize divine healing as do the Christian miracle churches.[8]

One interviewee serves as a Christian pastor at the head of a (non-miracle) church largely comprised of Africans from neighboring countries of anglophone (English-speaking) Africa. The pastor is from outside of Mozambique. This religious leader offers particular insights due to broader experience in Africa, leadership of the congregation, and a position as an insider/outsider in Mozambique. The pastor made a number of observations regarding the relationship between health and religion. First, the pastor thought that a higher percentage of people go to traditional healers in Mozambique than elsewhere in Africa. The pastor stated that a greater percentage of people went to *curandeiros* within their ministry in the poorer suburban areas of Maputo than in what is frequently termed the "cement city" or central city. Second, the pastor stated that Christians generally steer sick people directly to hospitals. The cleric said that in Burundi, for instance, the growth of Christianity has caused more people to go to hospitals than before. Finally, the pastor affirmed that modern medicine cannot cure spiritual problems, just physical ones. Taken together, observations from the minister convey a quite informed and pragmatic view of the role played by religion in health care.

Religion and health provision

Two Mozambican health specialists with World Vision put forward their belief that all of the religious groups in the country provided health care. These groups include Christians, Muslims, and Traditional Healers. The officials divided Christians into two categories on the basis of their views on health-care provision and health-seeking behaviors. These two categories, positive and negative, clearly carried value connotations for the officials. The "positive" churches helped the members know what to do when sick. This process included getting people to the clinic when illness strikes. The health specialists also showed openness to the involvement of organizations like World Vision in working with local community groups on health issues.

---

[8] Traditional healers in Mozambique, who will be covered in greater detail later in this chapter, are called by the Portuguese word *curandeiros* (pronounced KoorahnDAYroosh). In Portuguese, this word literally means "curers," although the *Dicionário Português/Inglês* translates the term into English much more negatively as "quack, witch doctor, charlatan."

World Vision, in contrast, had not talked with the miracle churches about health-related issues because "it is difficult." Miracle churches, they said, have a lot of money, media access, and influence on the government. The miracle churches are viewed much more negatively by the World Vision interviewees with respect to both faith and health. Practical and theological disagreements persist between the two church categories on God's response to prayer. The World Vision people believed that God does not always respond immediately to a person's prayer request (positive churches), but the miracle churches (negative churches) taught that "He does." This latter belief, the World Vision health specialists argued, tended to demoralize people who did not receive immediate answers to prayer. They presented one case that they knew of personally where a pastor at a miracle church told a Christian that he must actually believe in a different God because his prayer had not been answered immediately. On health provision, the World Vision interviewees indicated a "competition" between miracle churches and doctors.

The World Vision health personnel saw Muslims as very organized compared to Christians in terms of health provision. Muslims operate kindergartens, schools, madrassas, and charities for the poor. They noted that while Muslims access health clinics, there were relatively few Muslim doctors. Most doctors are Christians. Muslims, the World Vision interviewees thought, also tend to go to *curandeiros* more than Christians.

An administrator for the Presbyterian Church of Mozambique made a number of points on the provision of public health by religious organizations. These observations focus on the evolution of faith-based health care, along with how it is connected to education. First, the administrator noted that religious organizations and individuals providing health care is not new in Mozambique. The Presbyterian Church, for example, has been in Mozambique for 125 years, with about 200,000 members. Early missions from its inception and on to today have placed a strong emphasis on religious instruction, education, and health. In order to reach more rural areas, the Presbyterian Church also started clinics to assist the population in obtaining access to hospitals. Church leaders thought it impractical to teach people to pray for healing and then simply observe them going to the *curandeiros*. Thus, the Presbyterian Church instituted a policy of "prayer and clinic." The Presbyterian Church and school provided another leg in that it educated people in these spiritual and physical areas.

Second, the original vision and activities of the Swiss missionaries, who started the Presbyterian Church in Mozambique, affected the subsequent trajectory of the church. Missionaries and their followers founded a number of hospitals throughout the country, including the Central Hospital of Chamanculo. At independence, the new Marxist government (which was very strongly anti-religion) nationalized all of the Presbyterian health facilities in the country. The church, the administrator noted, would now like to get the hospitals and property back from the government. This Presbyterian administrator did admit that the church in general was too poor to financially support the number of hospitals that it had operated before nationalization.

Third, and finally, the missionaries and church emphasized the education of youth and adults. As a result of both education in general and knowledge of the Bible in particular, according to the Presbyterian administrator, they were far less likely to go to a *curandeiro* for medical assistance. All of these efforts worked to influence the health-seeking behavior of church members and the provision of health services by the church.

The Presbyterian administrator also noted that some non-traditional (ie not mainline) churches do provide health care. African Zionist churches (Ziones) emphasize a cure for illness but without recourse to hospitals. The term used to describe the Zionists is "Maziones," which is a Shangaan (the predominant language of Southern Mozambique) word for "Zionist people." This interviewee thought that the Maziones were trying to get people to go to them for healing instead of the *curandeiros*. However, like the *curandeiros*, the Maziones did not emphasize modern medicine.

An officer from USAID in Mozambique, with health-related responsibilities, had a more programmatic approach to the impact of religion on health provision and health-seeking behaviors. USAID likes to look more at the positive norms for religion and seeks to promote ways in which religion can encourage positive "health behaviors." On the USAID website, there is the Center for Faith Based and Community Initiatives that examines these issues. The USAID officer indicated that a number of USAID-sponsored organizations and programs involve religious groups. First is PIRCOM, an organization mentioned earlier in this chapter. That organization is a strong proponent of combating malaria. A second organization is Strengthening Communities Through Integrative Programming (SCIP). This organization has community programs with World Vision that looks at how to better facilitate service provision in clinics.

An official with Muslim Community: Humanitarian Action (Comunidade Muçulmano: Acção Humanitária) confirmed that Muslims also provided health care. Muslim doctors are at the Ministry of Health. The official said that Muslims also operate two clinics in Maputo, which are open to people of all faiths.

Religion and health-seeking behavior

Religious beliefs affect behavior among those seeking health care. A Ministry of Health official also spoke on religion and health-seeking behaviors. In terms of Christianity—which the official defined broadly—two churches "caused serious problems" in terms of health-seeking behaviors for the Ministry of Health: the IURD and Jehovah's Witnesses. The interviewee said the Jehovah's Witnesses adherents refused blood transfusions due to religious beliefs. This caused concern for children with severe malnutrition as some with serious cases needed blood transfusions to survive. The concern being expressed focused on saving the life of the child, despite the strong religious objections of the parents to a blood transfusion. Two options exist. One procedure is to send the parents out of the room and then secretly give the blood transfusion to save the child's life. The parents never knew that their child would get the transfusion. The medical staff realized that they did not have the permission of the parents but also did not want the child to die. In some cases, the parents said "no" and the child died. It remains a difficult decision for the medical staff in either case.

About the IURD, the Ministry of Health official expressed the greatest concern, saying that the church "delays" people seeking medical attention. This interviewee also added that people pay money for a tithe to the church to be cured. Thus, it is also quite expensive as medical care is generally not charged for. The official did not know about any studies made on the veracity of the healings via the IURD and added that no evidence existed that the miracles worked. The official thought that it might be a financial scam between the church and those who had been "healed." The tithes, donations, and size of the church allow it to be quite powerful. The interviewee said that the church is the largest in Maputo, one of the largest in Africa, and even has its own television channel in Maputo. The church just inaugurated a large building two months prior to the interview at a prime location in the capital city of Maputo.

The IURD is very influential in the community because of its size. The Ministry of Health official said that a key advantage is its job connections. The interviewee said that someone would show up and says he needs a job. The church will suggest calling someone about possible employment. He gets the job, but the person does not know that the IURD has already contacted the employer (a member of the church). The leaders will then cite this as an example of God working. The IURD also has schools that teach technical skills and nurseries for workers. The Ministry of Health official added that the IURD television programming says the following:

1. Leave modern medicine.
2. Leave *curandeiros*.
3. Be cured through the church.

The Ministry of Health had not, however, contacted the church to discuss their health-messaging concerns. "It is not easy talking to them," asserted the official, "because the church is organized and powerful." The Ministry of Health had, nonetheless, earlier asked the church to stop saying "throw away your HIV pills" as this would negatively affect the health status of the HIV-positive individual and foster HIV resistance to the antiretroviral drugs due to non-compliance with the drug regimen. The Ministry of Health official said that no change resulted in the health messaging in the programs about "throwing out the medicine" after talking to the church.

Officials from the IURD disputed the charge that they did not encourage their members to seek medical care in addition to prayer. The church is clearly able to influence the population with health messaging due to its size, technical sophistication, and financial resources. The main church building of the IURD is very large, imposing, and modern in appearance. The quality of its construction is quite high. The building contains a large and airy underground parking garage, bookstore, and substantial worship area.

A church service took place in the main assembly room during the interviewee's visit. The service was being filmed and broadcast on the cable channel. The man engaged in purported healing had been on television a few days earlier. The church services run non-stop throughout the day and part of the night. There were a number of people present. The denominational bookstore had a book available on the Brazilian founder of the IURD, Edir Macedo. The church had spread worldwide from its start in Brazil.

A leader from the IURD conveyed the church's position on miracles and medicine. This leader said that the church believed that if you have a physical ailment like a cut on the arm or malaria, you should go to a doctor for treatment. There may also be a spiritual problem requiring prayer even if the doctor fixes the problem. If, however, the doctor could not heal the patient, then it must be a spiritual problem that needed prayer to cure. The church official stated that some people thought the church activities to be a sham, but asserted that the IURD genuinely wanted to help people.

When asked about *curandeiros*, the leader from the IURD was quite negative about them: "They may want to do good or bad." He stated that the IURD only wanted to do what would be good for the person. The health messaging on this seemed pretty clear from the leader's comment that a Christian should never go to a *curandeiro*.

To better explain the activities of the church, the interviewee showed a copy of a newspaper-formatted newsletter on the IURD in Mozambique, entitled *Folha Moçambique* and dated August 29, 2010. One of the articles inside covered the issue of baptism. An excerpt from the article is as follows: "How do you know if your baptism was valid? After water baptism sorrow, rancor, resentments, envy, pride, evil eyes, jealousy, in sum, all that symbolizes the flesh and the world ought to disappear." This material indicates a "holiness theology" as a core belief in the church. The holiness movement originally arose among 19th-century Methodists such as John Wesley and emphasizes the ability to live a life free from voluntary sin due to a second work of sanctification that occurs through baptism and the Holy Spirit. The first work of spiritual regeneration relates to salvation from the consequences of sin for the believer, which is provided through the atoning death of Christ. This latter theological position, which emphasizes grace, would generally be considered an orthodox viewpoint among nearly all Christian denominations. The holiness movement has a more perfectionist position on the individual's ability to overcome sin in this life.

An IURD television program on healing and miracles presented clear health messaging that shaped the health-seeking behavior of viewers. The program had fairly good production quality—fast-moving stories and testimonials. The church used the slogan: "Where the miracle is something natural." Presenters emphasized "curing through bálsamo," or oil that is placed on a hurting area to help the pain. Testimonials showed people with physical ailments, not readily apparent, being cured. Two segments featured cases of two separate women, allegedly crippled in their legs, walking around after being prayed for by the pastor.

The pastor of the church speaking on the program seemed Mozambican in appearance and accent but pronounced the Portuguese word for health with a Brazilian accent "saúdjee," as opposed to the Portugal and Mozambique accent of "saúde," which is "saúduh". This apparently indicated the influence of Brazilian training on the leaders. During the program, the pastor said the following: "Doctors cannot heal ailments like malaria, headaches, and paralysis." A saying appeared from time to time on the screen: "Miracles that the science of medicine would desire." A verse from Jeremiah 46:11 was in the background and seemed to hold particular importance: "Go up to Gilead to get medicine, O virgin daughter of Egypt! But your many treatments will bring you no healing" (*Holy Bible* 2004). This is a form of health messaging that could discourage conventional health-seeking behavior among members of the congregation.

The church official with the Presbyterian Church of Mozambique also noted the impact of religion on health-seeking behaviors for Muslims. This interviewee presented an illustrative example among the largely Muslim coastal areas of the northern provinces of Nampula and Cabo Delgado. The Presbyterian official had become familiar with the area because he lived and travelled in Nampula for some years. Such rural communities are a mixture of traditional religion and Islam. (The official further noted as a later aside that there has been a marked increase in the use of *curandeiros* by Muslims in these regions.) Cholera broke out in the area. The government started a campaign to halt the epidemic and treat the sufferers. Medics showed up in the region as part of this campaign but people beat up the medics and vandalized their property. Unfortunately, some inhabitants of these rural zones thought that the medics had actually brought the cholera with them in order to kill members of the community.

Government officials at the Ministry of Health affirmed the fact that most Mozambicans went to both African Traditional Religion-style *curandeiros* and Western-style, modern medicine doctors. People go to the *curandeiros* to cleanse themselves spiritually before they visit the clinic. The illness could be a physical or mental manifestation of an underlying spiritual issue. More specifically, they want to make sure that the physical ailment has not been caused by a neighbor with bad intent or due to a punishment (castigo) for a personal failing. A *curandeiro* can be costly. In case of a serious illness, a sick Mozambican would go to the hospital fairly quickly. Finally, the government officials noted that there is an Association of Traditional Medics.

With respect to Islam and health-seeking behavior, a Ministry of Health official stated that polygamy is one area of concern. According to most common Islamic jurisprudence interpretations, Muslims are allowed more than one wife—with four being the permissible limit. The government in general is trying to discourage polygamy and passed a law making 18 the lowest legal age for marriage. Polygamy is associated with health-related problems for women, over and beyond early marriage. Despite tension over this particular issue, the director said that Muslims do nonetheless tend to send their sick to clinics.

Traditional and spiritual healing

Traditional healers, or *curandeiros*, remain a very important means of health-care delivery in Mozambique. Provision depends on geography. The area where people make most use of the *curandeiros* is in the rural zones. The Presbyterian leader called this the "*curandeiro* problem." This interviewee also noted that, sometimes, only one member of the family will go to a *curandeiro*. Other members of the family may not like that decision, so patronizing a *curandeiro* can cause rifts in the family. The Presbyterian leader cites disturbing examples of what is observed in the less developed central and northern parts of the country. The first example presented by that leader is as follows: a son will be sick and go to a *curandeiro*; the *curandeiro* will say his sickness is due to his mother; and the son will therefore kill the mother. It is unclear how common this practice is, but it is either rare or at least rarely reported. A second example is that a *curandeiro* may also tell someone with HIV that it can be treated with traditional medicine. This delays the person seeking treatment from modern medical clinics where they can receive antiretrovirals. Sometimes, the person dies as a result. Finally, access to health care via *curandeiros* can be expensive. Someone diagnosed with malaria pays 10 meticais (about 30 US cents) at the hospital for treatment. A *curandeiro* may charge up to the equivalent of a small goat, which costs about 1,500 meticais (USD52).

The Ministry of Health official, unsurprisingly given their role, sounded more positive about interaction of the Ministry of Health with traditional healers (*curandeiros*) in providing care for Mozambicans. The official said that, in Nampula Province (located in the north of the country), the government had been coordinating with traditional healers' associations to try to organize them to work closely with the Ministry of Health. This interviewee indicated positive responses from the *curandeiros*, who believe that they can help to improve the results of community health. The Ministry of Health official's goal is to work in parallel with such traditional healers. These healers are working out instances where those who are ill are sent directly to the government in cases of HIV, malaria, asthma, TB, cholera, and epilepsy. Other interviewees asserted that medical professionals can work with *curandeiros* to convey basic treatments. An example might be teaching a *curandeiro* to cool a child with a wet piece of cloth on the way to a clinic in the case of a fever.

Within this northern, very traditional, and rural part of the country, the Ministry of Health is working with *curandeiros* on nutritional issues due to the chronic malnutrition that is common there. The Ministry of Health official gave as an example teaching these healers to add dried and powdered cassava leaves to porridge to boost the iron content and powdered cashew nuts for protein. The Ministry of Health also employs a weight chart for each child, and during every visit, weighs the child to see if the weight is tracking appropriately. Finally, the official said with some pride, after Ministry of Health training programs in Nampula Province, *curandeiros* sent the government 900 cases of possible TB infection and 99% of these referrals were confirmed as being correctly identified by the *curandeiros*.

Epilepsy is traditionally seen as a spiritual matter due to the physical convulsions it entails. To explain such cases, *curandeiros* argue that, for example, the mother did not get the medicine required when her child was born (or the wrong type of traditional medicine) and the child has therefore subsequently developed convulsions. Now, as a result of this partnership with the government, many of the *curandeiros* with whom the Ministry of Health works will send the child to a clinic immediately if there are convulsions. Since there is no readily available cure for convulsions—anti-seizure drugs are expensive and out of reach for many—the *curandeiros* may attempt to heal them. Some epileptic patients do report feeling better after receiving traditional medicine, which the director said is fine with the Ministry of Health. In cases where the *curandeiro* expresses the need to attend to spiritual matters, the Ministry of Health encourages them to do that relatively quickly and then speed the sick patient to the clinic. The government also strongly discourages the practice of keeping the sick person in a room in the *curandeiro*'s house.

The Ministry of Health official indicated that the Traditional Medicine Institute understood that being a *curandeiro* is a source of income for an individual. If the *curandeiro* is not making money, they will not send the patient to the clinic. However, more positively, when *curandeiros* believe that they are receiving adequate compensation for spiritual assistance, they will cooperate and send patients to the clinic. The official also said that *curandeiros* can be expensive. A patient in Maputo may be charged USD30–100. A white person seeking help from a traditional healer in Maputo may be charged up to USD1,000, the official said. In rural areas, charges are lower because people are poorer. In certain rural areas, some people are too poor to pay for the services at all. The *curandeiro* may then ask for a daughter to be given as a wife for payment.

Overall, the Ministry of Health official seemed to envision a model of public health in which serious physical needs are attended to by modern medicine and emotional, mental, and spiritual needs by religious believers. This is pragmatic in a location greatly challenged for resources, such as poverty-stricken Mozambique.

Curandeiros, as already seen, remain a major source of health-care provision for Mozambicans. The World Vision health workers stated that Mozambicans rely on *curandeiros*, especially in the north of the country where the lack of roads and the rural nature of society make it difficult to walk very far. This is even more the case when the person is sick or pregnant. Sometimes, people go to the *curandeiros* first or alongside modern medicine. If the patient is sick or even dies, the question arises as to why. The *curandeiro* provides the justification. Thus, before going to the clinic, the person goes to the *curandeiro* to learn why he or she is sick. After that has been assessed, then the individual goes to the hospital or clinic, if available. In Maputo (again, in the more developed and central part called the "cement city"), people do not go as much to *curandeiros*. In the less developed suburbs (the so-called "cane city"), people do use *curandeiros*, but many who live there are actually recent migrants from rural parts of the country.

The World Vision personnel presented a similar approach to categorization for *curandeiros* as for Christians. There are two types of *curandeiros*: good ones and bad ones. They emphasized that—good or bad—a *curandeiro* is an "opinion leader." People follow their advice, even government officials. The bad ones have gone commercial and promote themselves through marketing campaigns. They are selling their services. Recently, many *curandeiros* from Nigeria, the Democratic Republic of the Congo, and Tanzania have moved to Maputo. Their charges are relatively expensive. *Cuandeiros* also specialize in the treatment of sexual problems, employment, and so on. Clients must pay or get no service.

Good *curandeiros*, by contrast, are located in the rural communities where people depend on them. Any medical care must come in that way. These *curandeiros* help the community and know their treatments. If a person cannot pay, the *curandeiro* will treat for little or nothing. They might even let a patient stay for free in a room in their house. The *curandeiro* might ask for some payment later as money comes available to the patient's family. Good or bad, *curandeiros* augment, but do not necessarily replace, modern medicine. In sum, a good *curandeiro* replaces modern medicine only when cures are not available, while a bad one competes with available, effective treatments.

Discussion of traditional and spiritual healing so far has focused on the large and diverse Christian community. An official with the Muslim Community: Humanitarian Action (Comunidade Muçulmano: Acção Humanitária) affirms that some Muslims also use *curandeiros*. He said that this is wrong in terms of the teachings of Islam. The person who goes to a *curandeiro* is healed but then gives glory to the man and not to God; this exults the man above God, which is wrong. The Muslim official stated that going to a faith healer was a cultural aspect of many Africans. Muslims, however, should go to doctors.

Evaluation of the role of religion in health care

Research in Mozambique permits an initial assessment of the relationship between religious beliefs and health-seeking behaviors. Interviews confirm the guiding principle that religious belief affects the delivery, procurement, and perception of health. Interviewees universally held that good health is necessary and that modern medicine is a means to that end. No matter the religious belief of the individual, all remained aware of the importance and efficacy of medical treatment. We found no real differences among Christians, Muslims, and followers of traditional African religious customs in this respect. Access to health care varies due to income and geography. Rural, remote, and poor areas are simply more challenging to serve. Religion also affects educational levels, with Christian groups, particularly those located in the southern region of the country, having higher educational levels than Muslims and culturally animist Mozambicans. Part of this is a legacy of the colonial era; the southern part of the country is more developed and Roman Catholic, while the northern part of the country is less developed and more animist and Muslim. The north is also less impacted upon by the legacy of the Portuguese educational system.

We did find that a religious world view tends to see health in a broader manner rather than simply physical. Clearly, one's health is also related to spiritual condition, though it is not always apparent to the individual how this is so. What differs markedly is the degree to which the physical, emotional, and psychological aspects of the individual remain separate from the spiritual. The more traditional Christian (and, as far as could be ascertained from the limited interviews, traditional Muslim) believes that the physical body may be healed distinct from an underlying spiritual cause. There may, however, may be an epiphenomenal spiritual cause of suffering that would require prayer.

Emerging churches and *curandeiros* share a very different understanding of the relationship between the spiritual and physical world. They see the physical, mental, and emotional spheres of an individual as being embedded within a larger spiritual sphere. One analogy might be the fruit that is embedded within Jell-O. The fruit represents the physical and other aspects of the individual and the Jell-O is the spiritual world. Thus, physical ailments are manifestations of a spiritual difficulty. The IURD and *curandeiros* thus focus on understanding the spiritual causes that heal the individual. Both groups received criticism that healing efforts had been ineffective, been inappropriate, delayed potential intake into a hospital, and been done for financial gain. Such groups, particularly the IURD, might say similar things about the medical profession.

The Ministry of Health tries to bridge the gap in mindsets by recognizing the financial requirements of the *curandeiro* profession while, at the same time, co-opting them. Their pragmatic formula is to use *curandeiros* as an early assessment tool for diseases, divert identified individuals to a hospital, and not concern themselves with the spiritual aspects of health. Ministry officials also accepted the "tax" resulting from an individual seeking help from both a *curandeiro* and a medical doctor. The Ministry of Health and other Christian groups also had more of a challenge with (co-opting) the emerging churches such as the IURD due to its size, sophistication, and power. These churches (for their part) are much less inclined to change their core theological beliefs to suit the needs and desires of the Ministry of Health.

There is also some competition between Christian churches and traditional healers on the nature of spiritual healing. The Christians interviewed acknowledged that some *curandeiros* wish to do well but thought that not all did. Serious theological differences exist over the source of the spiritual power. This seems to be less of a concern among Muslims, who are apparently more likely to be syncretistic. Overall, religious belief is important to individuals' world view and affects how they understand health-seeking behaviors. Clearly, other variables, such as education and rural versus urban location, influence health outcomes.

Processes and outcomes

Processes

This chapter focuses on the relationship between religious beliefs and health-seeking behaviors in Mozambique. Interview-based research confirmed the generalization from the academic literature that religious belief is important to individuals' world view and affects how they understand health-seeking behaviors. Religious belief affects the delivery, procurement, and perception of health. Clearly, there are other variables, such as education and rural/urban location, that influence processes pertaining to health. No matter the religious belief of the individual, all seemed aware of the importance and efficacy of medical treatment. On that point, no discernible differences emerged among Christians, Muslims, and followers of traditional African religious customs.

Religious beliefs did see health in a broader, more holistic, manner than physical processes. Mozambicans believe that one's health is also related to spiritual condition, though it is not always clear to the individual how this is so. What differed markedly among interviewees was the degree to which the physical, emotional, and psychological aspects of the individual remained separate from the spiritual. More traditional Christians believe that the physical body may be healed of some ailment without direct reference to an underlying spiritual cause. There may, however, may be an epiphenomenal spiritual reason that would require prayer. By contrast, the emerging churches and *curandeiros* shared a very different understanding of the relationship between the spiritual and physical worlds. They saw the physical, mental, and emotional spheres of an individual as being embedded within a larger spiritual sphere.

Efforts by the Ministry of Health to bridge the gap and cooperate with *curandeiros* are ongoing. More problematic to the Ministry is the relationship with mega-churches that claim the ability to perform miracles. The great power of these entities challenges the ability of modern medicine to reach their members as they are offered as alternatives to Western-style medicine. This is a problem over and above that posed by poverty.

From the standpoint of the Social Determinants of Health, the role of religion is confirmed strongly in this case. Religious beliefs are significant for consumption and faith-based entities are essential to provision with regard to health. The enduring story is one of demand exceeding the supply available from conventional, government-based outlets for health care. Some preference for faith-based health care obviously plays a role in determining tastes among the public. Mozambicans, all things considered, are holistic in their preferences and quite rational in tactics when it comes to health care.

Outcomes

This review begins with aggregate figures regarding change in the MDGs. It includes an assessment of the numbers to detect significant nuances with regard to women's health in particular.

With reference to MDGs 2 and 3 of achieving universal primary and secondary education by 2015, the Mozambique Country Report on the MDG Progress for 2010 showed a remarkable increase for primary enrollment between 1997 and 2008, from 22% to 77% and up to 81% thereafter (Ministry of Planning and Development, Government of Mozambique 2010: 34–38). The report points out that the highest attainment is in the southern region of the country, in Maputo Province. The rate of boys' enrollment in primary school is higher than for girls in all wealth quintiles, while most pronounced at lower wealth levels (2010: 38). Additionally, the male–female ratio is more extreme in rural areas. The Mozambique Country Report (2010: 38–39) also shows that the completion rate is highest in Maputo Province and, in general, there is a 20% difference between primary school completion between the lowest quintiles (72%) and highest (92%), even though education is free (2010: 39). In the secondary schools, the proportion is close to 1:1 for urban areas but about 0.75 for rural areas. As with the primary school enrollment figures, numbers for secondary school are explained most strongly by wealth differences, with the figures ranging from 0.43 to 0.58 (ie girls to boys) in the lowest wealth quintiles and the ratio being closer to 1 at the higher levels (2010: 48). Unlike the Ugandan report, that for Mozambique does not assess the rate of completion with reference to the MDG 2015 targets. It did show that girls are slightly more likely to be required to repeat a grade (at 59%) than boys (at 57%) (2010: 49).

Perhaps not surprisingly, the clustering of female illiteracy follows regional lines (as does primary and secondary school enrollment). In fact, Maputo region (south) reported a significantly higher attainment of literacy as compared to poorer central and northern provinces (Ministry of Planning and Development, Government of Mozambique 2010: 50–51). Nonetheless, the government reported that the levels of female illiteracy did decline from 66% in 2004 to 56% in 2009, with women disproportionately enrolled in adult literacy programs.

With regard to women's health laws, Mozambique surpassed, for instance, Uganda in 2014 and became one of the most liberal sub-Saharan countries on abortion. According to the *International Business Times*, a law passed in the summer of 2014 and signed by the president in December allows abortion for elective reasons in the first trimester

(12 weeks), extended up until 16 weeks in the case of rape (IBT 2014). The *International Business Times* article also mentioned the excessive maternal mortality rate in Mozambique, at 490 deaths per 100,000 live births. Additionally, it is known that those mostly at risk for unsafe abortion in Africa are teenagers. According to the Guttmacher Institute (2015), Mozambique is now somewhat similar to Ethiopia in terms of abortion law. Ethiopian law liberalized in 2005 to allow abortion not just in cases of maternal life or health, but also for fetal impairment, rape, incest, or inability to raise a child based on physical or mental infirmity (Guttmacher Institute 2015). This is due to work with the Pathfinder International foundation, a reproductive rights foundation. Pathfinder International began working with the international women's health coalition in 2011, recognizing that the existing law, which only allowed abortion in the case of threats to a woman's life or physical health, contributed to high rates of maternal mortality (Badiani 2016). In light of such ongoing problems, the governments of Canada and Sweden gave millions to Mozambique in 2017 to promote better family planning and safer abortion services (*Africa Review* 2017; York 2017).

Concerning MDG 4 (infant/child mortality), Mozambique reported in 2010 that it would "probably" meet the 2015 targets. Between 1997 and 2008, the under-five mortality rate decreased from 245 to 138 per 1,000 live births and the under-one mortality rate decreased from 143 to 93 during that same period (Ministry of Planning and Development, Government of Mozambique 2010: 56). The 2015 targets were 108 and 67, respectively. As with the other trends surveyed, Maputo City and Province performed the best (lowest mortality rate) on these scores (2010: 57). Child mortality is most related to malaria (42%), AIDS (14%), and pneumonia and diarrhea (each at 6%) (2010: 63).

With respect to MDG 5—maternal mortality and access to comprehensive reproductive care services (especially contraception)— the Mozambique Country Report (Ministry of Planning and Development, Government of Mozambique 2010: 67) claims that the maternal death reduction target of 250 per 100,000 by 2015 is "potentially" within reach. However, the country's figures of 692 such deaths per 100,000 in 1997 and 500 in 2007 would seem to argue strongly against that designation (2010: 67). The percentage of births occurring within the presence of skilled birth attendants rose from 44% to 55% during the same time period, with a 2015 goal of 66% (2010: 67). Data showed that the 15–30 population age group suffered 66% of the overall maternal deaths and, of course, in-hospital deaths were about one fifth to one sixth of those happening outside hospitals (2010: 68). Similar to Uganda, the vast majority of deaths (76%) are due to direct causes during birth, with the highest being uterine rupture (17%), hemorrhage (14%), eclampsia (13%), and sepsis (11%). AIDS appears as the most prevalent indirect cause of death (at 12%) (2010: 68). Similar to the other figures in this chapter, Maputo Province and City had the lowest rate of maternal mortality due to the highest rate of in-hospital births (2010: 69). Only 17% of attended births occurred in facilities with obstetric emergency care, with only 11% of the overall need met (2010: 72). Similar to Uganda, the constraints of location and hospital facilities (including sufficient personnel) strongly affect birth outcomes for mothers and babies.

The contraceptive use rate is surprisingly low when compared to Uganda, being about half, at 6% in 1997, 16% 10 years later, and with a 2015 target rate of only 34% (Ministry of Planning and Development, Government of Mozambique 2010: 68). Consistent with the discussion so far, poorer and rural families use more traditional methods of contraception (withdrawal and condoms), while urban and wealthier families (including those in Maputo) implement more modern methods such as chemical contraception (2010: 72–73). The Mozambique Country Report (2010: 73) notes that:

> facts such as inadequate management of the family planning programme, insufficient information and education of the population and deficient integration of men into the sexual and reproductive health policies/strategies ... may limit the expansion of the programme and meeting of the 34% target for contraceptive prevalence rate in 2015.

Indicative of the family-planning problems is that the individual average fertility rate showed virtually no change between 1997 and 2007, from 5.9 average children per woman to 5.8 (2010: 74). As mentioned earlier, access to, and awareness of, birth control varies by income and location. Mozambique is a largely rural country with relatively high levels of poverty and illiteracy, particularly in the northern region.

The Mozambique report is consistent with United Nations Children's Fund (UNICEF) and United Nations Development Program data showing that higher education rates for women yield better contraceptive, sexuality, and motherhood information and outcomes. For example, while 38% of girls without schooling had their first sexual intercourse experience before the age of 15, only 11% of girls who reach secondary school levels are in this category (Ministry of Planning and Development, Government of Mozambique 2010: 75).

The Mozambique report shows a low rate for the utilization of condoms (1%) among those using contraception, which helps to explain the high unintended pregnancy rate and the fact that AIDS prevalence rose from 9% in 2003 to 12% in 2008 (Ministry of Planning and Development, Government of Mozambique 2010: 78). In addition, the rate of infection among pregnant women aged 15–24 was quite high (at 13%) in 2003, the last year for which figures are available (2010: 78). Unlike most other figures, in which progressive change is shown in the urban areas, the government reported a higher rate of HIV/AIDS in the cities (2010: 79). Women are more likely to be infected than men (2010: 80). Thus, MDG 6 is unlikely to be met at any time close to 2015. Additionally, Mozambique is one of the 10 countries in sub-Saharan Africa comprising 81% of the infected population (Make Every Woman Count 2016: 67–70). The poor rate of condom use does not help sexually active people avoid HIV infection. Working with the UNAIDS Global Plan to eliminate new HIV infections among children by 2015, the US President's Emergency Plan for AIDS Relief (PEPFAR) and UNICEF had a positive response from the Mozambican government, which reduced new HIV infection among children by 75%. Uganda had an even higher reduction, at 86% (UNAIDS 2017).

Interviews conducted between 2010 and 2013 for the African Women's Decade Mid-Term Review show that "thirty three percent of women do not make the final decision on their own health care in Mozambique" (Make Every Woman Count 2016: 68). As discussed earlier, an unfortunate finding is that the contraceptive prevalence rate has gone down since 2008, to 12% from 16%. The proportion of attended births has risen to about 54% in 2011 (Make Every Woman Count 2016: 69). The fertility rate has decreased to about 5.2 births per woman in 2011—another positive development. Higher fertility rates are also associated with relatively early marriage. Mozambique, however, is still listed as one of the top countries for child marriage in the world, getting a rating of 10th according to World Vision (2017). As noted in the other two country chapters, child brides (ie those under 18) tend to have higher rates of obstructed labor leading to longer delivery time, which can result in the development of fistulas. This, in turn, means not being able to have a live birth at a later date. Thus, much work remains to be done with regard to protecting women from abusive practices that entail a lifelong legacy.

Reproductive rights in Mozambique, a related issue, are impacted upon by widespread religious beliefs regarding the sanctity of the unborn child or the one to be born. It is speculative, but perhaps the imperfect but relatively strong reproductive rights would constitute one of the few positive by-products of the Marxist regime, which stressed gender equality and thereby weakened the influence of faith-based entities that would tend to argue in the opposite direction. The relatively strong role played by multilateral foreign donor agencies in funding health care may also account for the more liberal policies regarding reproductive rights. At the same time, it is discouraging to see low rates of contraception use in rural areas in particular. This might be linked to the greater power of traditional values and the role of *curandeiros* in such locations. Polygamy, a practice restricted to Muslims and more traditional African culture, might also be playing some kind of role in limiting the use of contraception. Polygamy, with multiple sexual partners, may also foster the transmission of HIV/ AIDS. Mozambique does not legally recognize polygamy, but the practice itself is not illegal. A key problem associated with polygamy is the tendency for it to involve marriages among those who are too young, especially girls.

Finally, education-related outcomes (MDGs 2 and 3) show some asymmetry favoring boys over girls in terms of attainment in general and literacy in particular. Improvement in MDGs 4 and 5, concerning infant and maternal mortality, is clear to see, but, of course, there is still a long way to go.

Summary

Religion is an essential element of health care as a process in Mozambique—an affirmation of the point of view associated with the Social Determinants of Health. Perhaps the most amazing thing of all is how religious beliefs have persisted despite active efforts from a Marxist government over the course of decades toward elimination. Given the impoverished condition of Mozambique, help from religious entities in the provision of health care turns out to be quite valuable. Some variation exists among Mozambicans in how physical and spiritual elements interact with each other to create health, but there is no denying the essential nature of each. A key point of difference concerns Christians and Muslims, on the one hand, and emerging churches and curandeiros, on the other. While Christians and Muslims are well integrated with modern health provision, the latter are at the edges or even in conflict with the government system.

With regard to health outcomes, the story told by a review of the MDGs is mixed. MDGs 2 and 3, which focus on education as an element of health understood comprehensively, show positive change. Girls, however, lag behind boys in terms of grade completion and literacy. This may be due to families devoting scarce resources to education for boys based on the view of a greater likelihood of providing for the extended family. Infant and child mortality (MDG 4) has become better with time, but not much has changed with respect to maternal mortality (MDG 5). The outcome data suggest that religious entities are helping across the board in terms of health, but it is also the case that some associated beliefs are holding back progress in specific areas, such as family planning.

5

Ethiopia

Overview

This chapter focuses on religion and health in Ethiopia. The two basic questions motivating this study are answered to some degree through the research of this chapter: "What is the role of religion in the Social Determinants of Health?"; and "How is it connected to outcomes?"

Prior to moving into details of this case, it is helpful to provide an overview of what will be discovered along the way. Ethiopia is an ancient and significantly rural state. It did not experience colonization and remains quite poor—a sustained trait, with health care being an ongoing challenge. Over the last several decades, attention naturally concentrated on HIV/AIDS. State-created local organizations that focus on health care have existed for some time. However, they are limited in their reach and effectiveness. Faith-Inspired Institutions add significantly to health care for Ethiopians, who tend to be religious. Modern medicine exists alongside holy water, traditional birth attendants, and other aspects of non-Western treatment. The Consortium of Christian Relief and Development Associations is an umbrella organization that coordinates various faith-based efforts to provide health care. Its role is constructive as a rallying point for health care provided via civil society in Uganda. Women's health, however, stands out as a problem area, as revealed through a review of the Millennium Development Goals (MDGs) in the Ethiopian context. Ethiopia lags behind other states and religious beliefs and even institutions sometimes play a negative role. In an overall sense, religion plays an essential role in the provision and consumption of health for Ethiopia and the story is thus, for the most part, a positive one.

While it stands out as a low-income, developing country, Ethiopia is also an ancient and independent state. Ethiopia is a poor country even by African standards. According to United Nations (UN) data, in 2010 (the most recent year for which information is available), 36.8% of the population lived on less than USD1.25 per day (calculated in terms of purchasing power parity). Economic and political reforms have contributed to a significant drop in this figure, even though the same period saw a major increase in the country's overall population.

In 1995, for example, the comparable number had been 63.2%. Furthermore, wealth in the country is not evenly distributed. Ethiopia had a Gini coefficient of 39.1 in 2015, measuring a relatively low level of income inequality in the country, according to the World Bank.[1] This indicates, however, that more income equality exists in Ethiopia than in Mozambique and Uganda, the two other cases in the volume.

Primary research reported in this chapter is interview-based and pertains to contemporary Ethiopia with regard to the role of religion in health care. A research team with personnel from Pepperdine University, USC (the University of Southern California), and Addis Ababa University conducted interviews within the capital city and its nearby vicinity during May 2014.[2] Interview subjects included academics, government officials, and non-governmental organization (NGO) employees. Contacts from Worku Tefera, a doctoral candidate at the School of Public Health, Addis Ababa University, greatly facilitated interviews that might otherwise have been impossible. A list of those interviewed, along with professional affiliations and dates, appears in the Appendix (see p 197).

Prior research at the intersection of religion and health care in Ethiopia is quite limited. Studies tend toward survey research, with a focus on potential national patterns. The intended contribution here is at the individual level. A study of this kind, based on interviews, is unprecedented for Ethiopia and should produce valuable insights about the way in which religion factors into health care.

This chapter continues in four additional sections. The first conveys the context of Ethiopia in a panoramic and necessarily brief way. The second section summarizes existing research on religion and health care in Ethiopia. With a focus on faith-based provision and behavior vis-a-vis health, the third section conveys the interview material on processes. The subsections on processes include: (1) the general importance of religion; (2) religion and health provision; (3) religion and health-seeking behavior; (4) traditional and spiritual healing; and (5) an evaluation of the role of religion in health care. A further

---

[1] https://data.worldbank.org/indicator/SI.POV.GINI?end=2015&locations=ET& start=1995&year_high_desc=false

[2] The team included Patrick James, Robert Lloyd, and Worku Tefera. These team members, collectively speaking, possess overlapping expertise on Africa, health care, and religion. Tefera, a doctoral candidate in the School of Public Health, Addis Ababa University, is Ethiopian. Remarks from Tefera at interview sessions are occasionally inserted into that section of the chapter because he played a significant role in clarifying and elaborating on answers from interviewees.

subsection covers health outcomes. The fourth and final section passes along conclusions.

Context

Ethiopia is a state located in the Horn of Africa. Approximately twice the size of the US state of Texas, Ethiopia is landlocked and bordered by Djibouti, Eritrea, Kenya, Somalia, South Sudan, and Sudan. Much of the country consists of mountainous highlands associated with the Great Rift Valley of Africa. Ethiopia has a population of about one hundred million people, making it the second most populous country in Africa after Nigeria. The capital and largest city in Ethiopia is Addis Ababa, located in the geographical center of the country (CIA World Factbook 2016). Addis Ababa is also the headquarters of the African Union.

Over 84% of Ethiopians live in remote rural areas (Woldemicael and Tenkorang 2010: 989–990). Ethiopia is ethno-linguistically diverse, with 86 languages (Callaghan-Koru et al 2013; Ethnologue 2016b). These traits pose obvious challenges to development and national integration. Amharic is the official language in the country, with 27% of the population. Oromo has more speakers, with 34%, and is the official working language used in the Ethiopian state of Oromo. Somali is spoken by 6.2% of the population and is the official working language in the state of Sumale. Tigrigna is the official working language of the state of Tigray and is spoken by 6% of Ethiopians. Other languages are spoken by fewer speakers. English is the primary non-Ethiopian language used for business and schooling (CIA World Factbook 2016).

Mountains have played a key role in Ethiopian history. A "massive platform" at the center covers about one half of Ethiopian territory and functions as a great rift; Ethiopia's lowlands, in particular, have proven very difficult to integrate with the rest of the country (Markakis 2011: 23, 44). Terrain provides part of the explanation for political fragmentation but also a nearly unique trait within Africa: a history free from colonization. More than this, Ethiopia even defeated its would-be Italian conquerors in the era of high imperialism at the strongly memorialized Battle of Adwa in 1896. This battle stands as the first in which an African military force managed a victory against one from Europe as part of a military campaign (Shinn and Ofcansky 2004: 63–64).

While the Italians eventually defeated the Ethiopians led by Emperor Haile Selassie, with occupation ensuing from 1936 through 1941, the state that emerged from that experience took a different form. Italian occupation, put simply, facilitated the centralization of authority when Selassie regained power (Markakis 2011: 112–114). Selassie's rule lasted until the Dergue (often shortened to the Derg, which means "Committee") deposed him in the revolution of 1974. "While radical Marxism was its avowed ideology," observes Markakis (2011: 161), "Ethiopian nationalism and a commitment to the nation-state project was the revolution's driving force." The Dergue regime, led by military officers, pursued central dominance and attempted to gain support through the nationalization of land, which had been held overwhelmingly by the elite (Markakis 2011: 181). In an overall sense, however, Dergue efforts toward integration failed, and ethnic and regional divisions remained strong, and even became the basis of a successful revolution. A coalition of rebel forces—the Ethiopian People's Revolutionary Democratic Front, the Eritrean People's Liberation Front, and the Oromo Liberation Front—overthrew the Dergue. Conflict in Eritrea became especially intense and, as a result of a wide range of problems, the regime fell from power in 1991. As part of a pre-revolutionary agreement, the Ethiopian People's Revolutionary Democratic Front led Eritrea to independence in 1993 and left greater Ethiopia. At that time, Ethiopia became a landlocked state.

With the 1995 Constitution of Ethiopia, the state transitioned into a *de jure* multiparty regime for the first time in its history. Ethiopia is an ethnic-based federal system with a parliament (Polity 2010). Following the state's inauguration, Freedom House ranked contemporary Ethiopia as "partly free" from 1995 to 2010. However, it has been rated as "not free" since, despite the continued holding of elections. In 2015, the Ethiopian People's Revolutionary Democratic Front won 95% of the seats and its allies the remaining few. The regime is also rated as fairly corrupt; with a score of 33 out of 100, Ethiopia ranks 111 among 177 states assessed for the Corruption Perceptions Index (Transparency International 2014). Transfers of power after respective elections have not brought about controversy.[3]

From an economic point of view, Ethiopia has been a mixed story over the years. Following years of weak performance, economic growth has recently been quite strong. Decades of war over Eritrea's independence caused injury and death, along with worsened economic conditions (Woldemicael and Tenkorang 2010: 990). Ethiopia also suffered from a significant and prolonged drought in the mid-1980s. Nonetheless, more recently, Ethiopia may be viewed as one of Africa's

---

[3]   Prior to the 2015 elections, many political opponents had been rounded up by the government (Freedom House 2016).

"best performing economies," with a growth rate of 10.6% from 2003/2004 to 2010/2011 (Ethiopian Civil Society Health Forum 2013: 1). This trend continues as it has had an average growth rate of 10.47% from 2010 to 2016 (calculated from World Bank: Ethiopia 2016). Gross domestic product (GDP) is close to USD30 billion. Yet, the literacy rate and life expectancy are estimated as 29.8% and 58.12 years, respectively (Transparency International 2014). Most Ethiopians remain poor.

Contemporary Ethiopia, in terms of its religious make-up, features about 50% Eastern Orthodox, 33% Muslim, 18% Protestants, and 3% "followers of traditional religion" (Central Statistical Agency [Ethiopia] and ICF International 2012: 3–4; Brown and James 2015). Table 5.1, which shows religion by district, reveals that the population is not uniform in terms of its distribution on a geographic basis. Among the 10 districts, the modal categories are as follows: five are Muslim; three are Ethiopian Orthodox Church; and two are Protestant. This pattern is interesting in light of the statistical distribution for Ethiopia as a whole, within which the Orthodox Church is at one half of the population. It appears from the district-based data that Muslims and Protestants are more geographically concentrated in comparison to members of the Orthodox Church.

The centrality of Christianity and Islam to Ethiopian life is reinforced through national holidays connected to the Eastern Orthodox Church and Islam (Shinn and Ofcansky 2004: 208–210). Some history of violence exists regarding Christians and Muslims. A war of conquest occurred in early modern times, with forced conversion to Islam among many Christians and others in the kingdom. Christian dominance, however, took hold over the long term, with religious adherence quite important throughout Ethiopian life and Muslims in lower status (Markakis 2011: 32–34).

However, during the time of the Dergue, the Ethiopian Evangelical Church, Mehane Yesus, became its most visible target as the regime attempted to suppress religion. Their efforts, however, resulted in failure. Ironically, a religious revival occurred during the Dergue era, with "many more converts to Christianity than to scientific Marxism at this time" (Markakis 2011: 187). The legacy of the anti-religious Dergue is a national holiday on May 28, when the *fall* of that regime is celebrated each year.

What about the role of religion in government and society today? A sense of balance emerges regarding religion and the state—neither advocacy nor suppression. The preamble of Ethiopia's constitution "includes the objective of living without religious discrimination" (Fox

Table 5.1: Religion by district for the population of Ethiopia

Religion	Ethiopia	Afar	Amhara	Benishangul-Gumuz	Gambella	Harari	Oromiya	Somali	SNNPR*	Tigray
Orthodox	43.5	3.9	82.5	33.3	16.8	27.1	30.4	0.6	19.9	95.6
Protestant	18.5	0.7	0.2	13.5	70.1	3.4	17.7	0.1	55.5	0
Catholic	0.7	0	0	0.6	3.4	0.3	0.5	0	2.4	0.4
Muslim	34	95.3	17.2	45	4.9	69	47.5	98.4	14.1	4
Traditional and other	3.3	0	0.1	7.6	4.9	0.2	3.9	0.9	8.2	0
Total region pop	73,750,932	1,390,273	17,221,976	784,345	307,096	183,415	26,993,933	4,445,219	14,929,548	4,316,988

Note: * Southern Nations, Nationalities, and Peoples' Region

Source: Government of Ethiopia, Central Statistical Agency – Ministry of Finance and Economic Development, "Population and Housing Census of 2007," Table 3.3 Population by Religion, Sex, and Five-Year Age Groups: 2007, p 109. Available at: http://catalog.ihsn.org/index.php/catalog/3583

2008: 269). Article 11 declares that there is no state religion. Article 27 provides "detailed protection for religious freedom," but rights can be limited under some conditions, for example, "to ensure the independence of the state from religion." On the one hand, political parties based on religion have been banned from 2003. On the other hand, defamation against religious leaders is a crime (Fox 2008: 269). The overall story of religion and the state today is one of an effort toward maintaining a balance.

With regard to health care, major efforts toward the development of a modern medical system began after the Second World War. Despite help from the World Health Organization and the UN Relief and Rehabilitation Administration, a truly national health-care infrastructure remained elusive (Slikkerveer 1982: 1861). Programmatic change began soon after the new democratic regime replaced the Dergue in 1993. Launched in 1993, the National Health Policy led to the Health Sector Development Programs that started in 1998. The Health Sector Development Programs "respond to a number of health issues experienced by the country, including increasing the health coverage and improving the quality of health services for rural and urban Ethiopia" (Ethiopian Civil Society Health Forum 2013: 1).

The Ethiopian Civil Society Health Forum (2013: 2) provides an overview of the system today. Ethiopian health service delivery is organized into a three-tier set-up, which is characterized by a first level of a Woreda/District health system comprising a primary hospital (with a population coverage of 60,000–100,000 people), health centers (15,000–25,000 population), and their satellite health posts (3,000–5,000 population), which are connected to each other by a referral system. The Essential Health Service Package contains five components: "family health services; communicable disease prevention and control services; hygiene and environmental health services; health education and communication services; and basic curative care and treatment of major chronic conditions" (Ethiopian Civil Society Health Forum 2013: 2). Thus, on paper, Ethiopia shows the workings and priorities of a modern health system.

Results in health, however, lag behind stated priorities. Ethiopia ranks 173 out of 187 states on the UN Human Development Index, partially because of "a high rate of maternal mortality and the existence of regional disparities in basic health service delivery" (Ethiopian Civil Society Health Forum 2013: 1; see also Birhanu et al 2012: 162). Ethiopia is among the 10 highest states in the world for neonatal deaths, with an estimated 122,000 per year (Callaghan-Koru et al 2013: 2).

Major communicable diseases include HIV/AIDS, tuberculosis, and malaria.

Ethiopia's major health problems remain largely preventable (Ethiopian Civil Society Health Forum 2013). About 80% of diseases are related to "personal and environmental hygiene, infectious diseases and malnutrition" (World Health Organization, Regional Office for Africa 2013: xiii). An especially unfortunate example of a preventable malady is female genital mutilation, which persists at high rates and puts an additional burden on Ethiopia's health system (Yirga et al 2012: 46, 51).[4]

Perhaps at least in part as a result of Health Sector Development Programs, Ethiopia's Human Development Index moved from 0.275 (2000) to 0.396 (2012) (Ethiopian Civil Society Health Forum 2013: 1). It is clear that things are moving in the right direction. The Ethiopian Civil Society Health Forum (2013: 2, 3, 5) summarizes progress in health for Ethiopia:

- infant and under-five mortality decreased by 39% and 47%, respectively, between 2000 and 2011;
- HIV/AIDS among adults has dropped to 1.5% in 2010/2011 in comparison to the MDG target of 2.5%;
- the percentage of children sleeping under insecticide-treated nets increased from 3% (2005) to 33% (2010/2011); and
- the national tuberculosis detection and treatment success rate is estimated to have reached 63% and 88% in 2011/2012, respectively.

Ethiopia's public sector has worked in tandem with organizations from civil society to achieve these results. Documents from entities such as the Ethiopian Catholic Secretariat Health and HIV/AIDS Unit (2009), Ethiopian Civil Society Health Forum (2013) and World Vision Ethiopia (2014) show considerable work in progress. Box 5.1, from World Vision Ethiopia (2014), provides an example of a major project, in this instance, focusing on water supply.

---

[4]   For a strongly worded condemnation of female genital mutilation on religious grounds, consult the Catholic Bishops' Conference of Ethiopia (2013: 5, 20, 23).

Box 5.1: Spring of Life at Mount "Yekashe" for 25,000 People

Since 2011, World Vision Ethiopia has been working on a gravity-fed water supply project to provide adequate and safe water to more than 25,000 people in SNNPR at Muhurena Aklil District. The source of water, "Yekashe" spring, has the potential discharge to supply more than 40,000 people, including multiple uses. This "Spring of Life" was flowing for centuries while the people living in the area, including the district capital Hawariat (Aposte), suffered to get safe water. They were subjected to waterborne diseases and had to walk for hours over difficult terrain to fetch water. This drudgery primarily fell to women and children, which contributed to gender inequality and school dropout in the area. To date, 80% of the work has been completed, with 186 water taps providing access to safe water for about 20,500 people.

Source: Adapted from World Vision Ethiopia (2014: 3).

Ethiopia's context, to sum up, contains elements of uniqueness as well as traits in common with other states in sub-Saharan Africa. Like only one other state on the continent, it escaped colonization.[5] This, in part, reflects Ethiopia's difficult terrain, which also poses ongoing challenges to national unity and standards for policy. Like many other states on the continent, Ethiopia is a relatively recent convert to multiparty elections, with the veneer of democracy, after a long life under clearly autocratic rule. Ethiopia is poor even in comparison to other African states and suffers from significant health problems, many of which are preventable. Attention now turns to what is known so far about religion's role in health on the basis of prior scholarship pertaining to Ethiopia.

Religion and health care in Ethiopia: what we know so far

With a focus on rural health and the utilization of traditional healers, Slikkerveer (1982) offered a prescient assessment of Ethiopia more than three decades ago. For a state with great need, Slikkerveer (1982: 1860–1861) saw value in an "integrated approach" and "pluralistic view" regarding traditional and modern medicine. His research focused on the Hararghe province, the largest in Ethiopia. The traditional medical systems he identified include "macro-religious practices and the application of medicinal plants, often in combination with local

---

[5]   However, Italy did occupy Ethiopia during the Second World War. The other African country not considered to have been colonized is Liberia.

home remedies" and reflect syncretism of mystical and pragmatic beliefs (Slikkerveer 1982: 1862, 1863). The cast of characters in the traditional system entails "different categories of mystic and religious healers, herbalists, astrologers, bone-setters, traditional birth attendants and other functionaries," accounting for an estimated 45.6% of total patient visits (Slikkerveer 1982: 1865). At the time of the study, administrators and planners in the modern system tended to be skeptical about the potential contributions of traditional healers (Slikkerveer 1982: 1868). This study, with its call for a more integrated approach toward traditional and modern medicine, rings true today.

More recent studies of Ethiopia reveal a shift in attention to HIV/AIDS. Abebe et al (2003: 1836) report findings from a study of HIV prevalence among 72,000 men recruited in 1999 and 2000. The main result, in connection to religion, is that the rate of HIV is higher for Orthodox Christians than Muslims.

Molle et al (2008) focus on religious belief and sexual activity among religious and non-religious youth. The study found no difference between the sexual activity of religious and non-religious youth in a predominantly Muslim area of Ethiopia. "Although virginity norms help delay age at sexual debut among rural Ethiopian youth, and thus reduces vulnerability to sexually transmitted infections and HIV infection," Molle et al (2008) observe:

> vulnerability among females may increase after marriage due to unprotected multiple risky sexual behaviors by spouses. The use of preventive services, such as Voluntary Counseling and Testing VCT before marriage and condom use in marriage should be part of the HIV/AIDS prevention and control strategies.

The effects from religion can vary by age and context vis-a-vis sexual activity.

Woldemicael and Tenkorang (2010) investigate maternal health-seeking behavior. Data from the Ethiopian Demographic and Health Survey (Central Statistical Agency [Ethiopia] and ORC Macro 2006) are used for quantitative analysis of maternal health-seeking behavior as measured by the index. Through the use of factor analysis, these scholars create an index that consists of patient access to tetanus injection, antenatal care, and delivery care. While numerous demographic variables are included in the research design, of most interest here are results pertaining to religion. The rank order among major religious groupings with respect to the index is as follows:

Christians, traditionalists, Muslims (Woldemicael and Tenkorang 2010: 993, 994). Differences are significant and reveal that Muslims, in particular, lag with respect to accessing modern facilities when it comes to maternal health-seeking behavior.

Berhanu (2010: 241) studies the "beliefs, attitudes and experiences" of people living with HIV/AIDS at four holy-water sites. The study includes "in-depth interviews and key informant interviews to address the stated research questions" at four of 120 churches in Addis Ababa (Berhanu 2010: 245). All of those interviewed used holy water and "spoke of its healing power"; Berhanu (2010: 248, 256) concludes that "the situation demands more work at the grassroots level to allow the belief systems of individuals including priests and other servants of the church to include HIV ART [Anti Retro Virus] medication as beneficial."

With a focus on perceptions and practices, Ragunathan et al (2010) produce a study of traditional health practitioners. Research took place in Dembia district, Koladiba town, located in the North Gondar zone of the Amhara National Regional Government. The study included 23 modern health practitioners and 19 traditional health practitioners. Findings can be summed up as follows: (1) 60% of modern practitioners believe that traditional healing is important for maintaining sufficient health care; and (2) 94.7% of traditional practitioners saw their type of service as accepted by the community. While the results point toward the existence of goodwill between the two types of practitioners, it should be noted that most did not report interacting with each other. Moreover, the traditional system is known to incorporate some harmful beliefs and practices; education for traditional healers therefore becomes a priority (Ragunathan et al 2010).

Birhan et al (2011: 2) study the role of traditional healers, defined as "a [non-Western] educated or lay-person who claims ability or a healing power to cure ailments," in the health-care system of Addis Ababa. Birhan et al (2011: 2, 3) interviewed 10 traditional healers (seven of whom identified as Orthodox Christians), along with 306 patients, and found this option to be the first choice in health care for 172 (56.2%). Patients cited a number of reasons for why they visited a given traditional healer: previously treated and cured; efficacy; and dissatisfaction with, or cost of, modern medicine. All of the traditional healers used both dry and fresh plants for the preparation of remedies and 70% "identified diseases and causes of illness by history-taking and physical diagnosis" (Birhan et al 2011: 3). Most patients reported preferring traditional over modern health clinics, with a belief in greater efficacy that may reflect belief and culture (Birhan et al 2011: 5).

Unfortunately, the study revealed that traditional healers and modern health workers lacked motivation to collaborate and communicate with each other (Birhan et al 2011: 5).

Birhanu et al (2012) focus on patients' perception of empathy on the part of those treating them at health centers. The study is the first of its kind for Ethiopia and possibly even for Africa. Data for quantitative analysis came from a cross-sectional study, from December 29, 2009 to January 21, 2010, in the West Shewa Zone (Birhanu et al 2012: 162). The study reports results of the assessment of health worker empathy by patients in connection with various factors: socio-demographic, institutional, interpersonal, and others. Of key interest here is the association with the patient's religion; consistently, those affiliated with the Ethiopian Orthodox Church perceived greater empathy from health center workers.[6] When patients classified as "others" are looked at more closely, the perceived empathy score is most notably lower for those who follow an indigenous Oromo religion (Wakafena) (Birhanu et al 2012: 163, 165, 166).

Although many may not consider female genital mutilation a form of health treatment, its use is clearly impactful for women's well-being. This practice is the subject of a study by Yirga et al (2012) at the district level. The research team conducted house-to-house interviews in the Kersa Demographic Surveillance and Health Research Center field site. The town of Kersa is located in South-Eastern Ethiopia, specifically, within the Arsi Zone of the Oromia Region. The survey reached 858 women of reproductive age (15 to 49 years) from January to February 2008 (Yirga et al 2012: 47). The performance of female genital mutilation turned out to be quite frequent, with the percentage reaching a reported 94% in one rural area (Yirga et al 2012: 49). While the results do not include data on religion, it is noteworthy that: (1) traditional healers, using unhygienic procedures, performed about 75% of the reported instances of female genital mutilation; and (2) the research team calls for in-depth study of "cultural and religious" reasons for the practice (Yirga et al 2012: 52, 50). It is strongly implied by the study that traditional medicine, without connection to the modern variety, can produce harmful results.

Tilahun et al (2012), in a study looking at how attitudes might impact health-care delivery, investigate the attitudes of health workers regarding sexual and reproductive health services for unmarried adolescents. The research team implemented a cross-sectional survey that reached 423

---

[6] Protestants, in comparison to the Orthodox, perceive lower empathy, but the difference is not statistically significant (Birhanu et al 2012: 163, 166).

out of 1,704 health workers at two hospitals and 83 health centers in Eastern Hararghe (ie Oromia Region). Statistical analysis of worker attitudes does not reveal any connection with religion, measured as Muslim, Christian, or others (Tilahun et al 2012: 5). Interestingly enough, most health workers "had a positive attitude toward provision of sexual and reproductive health services to unmarried adolescents" (Tilahun et al 2012: 6). This points toward a trend in the direction of secularism within public health provided by the government.

Others have studied the question of why so many women in Ethiopia prefer home births. Shiferaw et al (2013) address this in a study utilizing survey research. With the predominantly rural area of Kembatta-Bembaro as the setting, Shiferaw et al (2013: 2) conducted a cross-sectional survey that included women from 15 to 49 years of age, the standard childbearing years. The research team also carried out in-depth interviews and group discussions. The data collectively confirm a preference for traditional birth attendants even with the availability of modern medical facilities and trained personnel. Greater empathy and respect in the traditional setting, as compared to modern facilities, came up as a major theme. Responses also draw attention to communication problems concerning access that discourage the seeking out of modern facilities, which might be closed at times of greatest need.

Callaghan-Koru et al (2013) investigate newborn care practices at home and in health facilities. Teams of interviewers collected data from four regions from January 4 to 27, 2012. Central results of the study are that: (1) women tended to deliver their babies at home; and (2) "the majority of women made one antenatal care visit to a health facility, but less than half made four or more visits" (Callaghan-Koru et al 2013: 6). While the demographic data collected by the research team included information on religion, this did not play a role in the statistical tables, which focused on very fine-grained information about health practices. Results from the study do point to the persistence of traditional healing as the preferred choice, which, in turn, is associated, in all likelihood, with religiosity.

While of high quality, studies located in the triangle of religion, health care, and Ethiopia are relatively few in number. What, then, can be said of the research in place already?[7] Four cover women's health (ie three maternal and one on female genital mutilation), two focus

---

[7] Additional studies on health care in Ethiopia might be included (eg Welle [2014] on rural water and the MDGs), but these tend to lack even a minimal connection to the role of religion.

on traditional healing, two examine health workers, and one looks at youth sexuality. The primary method across these studies is survey research. Some interviews are conducted, but results are conveyed, for the most part, through statistical tables. The studies carry out aggregate data analysis as opposed to evidence that would bear more directly on causal mechanisms. Thus, a shift toward interview-based research, to complement the breadth of existing research with further depth, seems in order.

Faith-based health provision and behavior: preliminary findings from interviews

The general importance of religion

Whether in response to a query or spontaneously, interviewees affirmed the importance of religion among Ethiopians. An official with the Ethiopian Evangelical Church observes that "Ethiopians are religious people." From the Ethiopian Catholic Secretariat, a member adds that "people believe in religion," and a professor from the School of Public Health, Addis Ababa University, emphasizes that religion is important. Other interviewees began their remarks in much the same way.

During a group meeting at the Consortium on Christian Relief and Development Associations, one participant asserted that "97% of the population is religious."[8] Something close to totality is affirmed for religion as a factor in Ethiopian life among various other interviewees as well. "Churches," according to a doctor affiliated with the Ethiopian Catholic Church and Save the Children, "are seen as providers of spiritual guidance." The doctor adds that religion is "a big thing." A professor from the School of Social Work, Addis Ababa University, mentioned a Coptic Orthodox background and currently identifies as an Evangelical. In addition, the professor worked at World Vision for six years in areas that included child development and rights. Religion,

---

[8]   Given the substantial attendance at the Consortium on Christian Relief and Development Associations meeting, in most instances, it proved impossible to associate a given participant with specific remarks. For that reason, speakers at this meeting are generally identified as "Consortium on Christian Relief and Development Associations interviewee." Along with several others, the following entities had representatives at the Consortium on Christian Relief and Development Associations: Christian Aid, the Ethiopian Evangelical Church Mekane Yesus Development and Social Services Commission, Ethiopian Orthodox Church Development and Inter-Church Aid Commission, and the Ethiopian Civil Society Health Forum.

based on his experience, is central to "identity and value formation." Thus, regardless of the source—whether a person is from a religious organization and therefore possibly biased in favor or someone else— the message about the centrality of faith is the same.

Affirmation of the full range of beliefs noted in the overview— Christianity, Islam, and traditional—pervades the interview material. For example, a professor at the School of Social Work, Addis Ababa University, observes that Christianity "goes back to the time of Enoch" (ie an ancestor of the biblical Noah), with Ethiopians reading and even memorizing passages of the Bible even prior to comprehension of its contents. The proportion of Ethiopians following traditional beliefs, according to an official from the Ministry of Health, is "significant." The professor just noted, who grew up in an Islamic region, affirmed its importance as well.

Religion plays an essential role in Ethiopian culture. This point is reinforced by a series of assertions from a participant at the Consortium on Christian Relief and Development Associations meeting: religious leaders have "power and acceptance" within their community. This is true despite oppression during the Dergue regime, which attempted to turn Ethiopia into a purely secular state. Ethiopian nationalism, favored by the Dergue, included a *religious* identification among the populace despite efforts to make it otherwise. This tactic on the part of the Dergue reflected a long history of religious faith among Ethiopians. Along such lines, Tefera observed that "long-standing beliefs are not erased by relatively short-term efforts." Religion, asserts an official from the Ethiopian Orthodox Church, "will be there" and constitutes "a basic human tendency." Thus, religion produces values and Redie sees cultural aspects of religion as essential.

Illustrations of the important role played by religion in everyday existence abound among remarks offered by interviewees. The professor from Addis Ababa University asserts that Ethiopians see religion as central to life. Saints, for example, play a key role—days of the week are named after them.[9] The professor adds that Ethiopia is mentioned many times in the Bible. The connection of Ethiopia with the Christian faith is manifested throughout the culture via icons and behavior. This interviewee offers a wide range of examples: baptism is the norm among Ethiopian Christians and wearing a cross is common.

---

[9] For example, in Argobba, a Muslim region, weekdays are named for saints: "'Tuesday': *nur ahusin* (Arg.), a Moslem saint born on Tuesday, worshipped in southern and western Ethiopia; and 'Wednesday': *abdeqader* (Arg.), a Moslem saint" (Leslau 1961: 62).

Pictures of Saint George are pervasive in cars. Fasting is common and not just during Lent or Ramadan. Adherence to fasting is strict in rural areas—even nine hours per day.

Christianity's central role in Ethiopian culture is confirmed when looking at social deviance as well as mainstream culture. A doctoral candidate at the School of Social Work, Addis Ababa University, had police experience prior to pursuing a PhD and offered a few recollections from that time. While in lock-up, criminal suspects routinely would ask for access to their "holy father." The doctoral student possesses ongoing links with corrections and criminal justice and sees the role of religion as quite prominent throughout the system. This interviewee notes that evangelists work persistently in prisons. Priests and other religious figures, moreover, play a role in promoting peace. The doctoral student sees that as especially true in the countryside; emphasis is placed on their role in "reconciliation." This interviewee did not volunteer specific details, but the promotion of inter-faith dialogue as a principal activity among religious leaders could easily be inferred from their remarks.

What about government and politics as related to religion? The Ethiopian state, as it turns out, contrasts with society, within which religion is crucial. An official from the Ethiopian Orthodox Church observes that "politicization of religion is minimized in Ethiopia." No textbook on religion, adds the professor just mentioned, "exists in the schools." Instead, the professor notes, public "schools are secular," but a tradition of mutual religious respect is "installed in students." (Madrassas and mission schools are also in operation.) This middle ground, manifested directly in the state's educational system, may reflect the society's religiosity in tandem with an imperative to manage potential conflict.

Although a tradition of mutual respect is part of Ethiopian society, it can sometimes be a point of contention (if not treated just right). Consider, along those lines, the observations of another professor from Addis Ababa University: the role of religion is "a very sensitive thing." When interviewed by TV Africa about waterborne diseases for a Muslim audience, the professor recalled putting an emphasis on science, not religion or politics. When on TV, the professor claims that "if I get into religion, it will be an offense." The professor implied that a Muslim can talk about scientific aspects of health care, but not in connection to *religious* beliefs and cleanliness as put forward by Islam. These observations reaffirm the idea that the Ethiopian government is seeking to keep religion separate from the state.

While excluded from the state, religion pervades Ethiopian society and interviewees identify that as important in a broad sense for health care. One professor provides a point of departure for such a discussion by noting that Ethiopia's religious culture can quite easily come into conflict with the secular West. An official from the Ethiopian Catholic Secretariat sees the modern world as affecting Ethiopia's culture "too fast," with change coming rapidly toward the individual. "African cultures," as one Consortium on Christian Relief and Development Associations meeting participant observes, "are different from the West." USAID (The United States Agency for International Development) (and Britain's parallel entity, the Department for International Development), from the point of view of many religious Ethiopians, tries to "force" the acceptance of homosexuality. According to the Consortium on Christian Relief and Development Associations meeting participant, this claim recalls Clinton-era conflict over teaching about the use of condoms. Put simply, there is an ongoing "clash of Western culture with faith/African cultures" because "Africans do not accept homosexuality." While some European churches even permit same-sex marriage, people of faith in Africa tend to look at things differently.

Several points emerge from the interviews with regard to the role of religion in Ethiopia. In a word, there is a strong consensus that religion is important to life in general. Religion shapes Ethiopian identity. It is also connected to the culture. Interviewees provided numerous illustrations of how religion matters a great deal in everyday life. The way in which the religiosity of Ethiopia conflicts with the secular world, notably, in encounters with the West, is apparent as well.

Religion and health provision

With regard to provision, discussion begins with a brief overview of government activity in order to provide a context for the discussion of faith-based activities. A review of the historical background will affirm long-standing involvement among religious entities. Contemporary efforts of Faith-Based Organizations in the health sector are extensive; their activities are covered in turn. This review is followed by a discussion of how the government and religious sectors are connected to each other. The overall character of religious provision is summed up as holistic in nature.

While it is beyond the scope of this study to focus on government provision in detail, visits to the Ministry of Health and one of the government health centers proved highly informative. The Ministry of Health shows high awareness of the key problems in public health.

Box 5.2, for example, displays the Ministry of Health's objectives and strategic plan regarding the mother-to-child transmission of HIV. The plan contains highly specific information that reveals a grasp of the situation and commitment to progress.

Box 5.2: "Federal Republic of Ethiopia, Ministry of Health, Elimination of Mother to Child Transmission of HIV (e-MTCT) Strategic Plan (2013–2015)"

Outcome Targets by 2015

1. Reduce the incidence of HIV in reproductive age group by 50%
2. Reduce the unmet need for FP to 10% among all women
3. Increase deliveries attended by skilled birth attendants to 62%
4. Increase proportion of deliveries of HIV positive women that receive HAART to 90%
5. Increase proportion of HIV exposed infants who receive ARV prophylaxis to 90%

Objectives of e-MTCT strategic plan

1. Improve community ownership through strengthening of Health Extension Program and Health Development Army to create demand and increase utilization of MNCH and e-MTCT of HIV services
2. Improve equitable delivery of quality integrated MNCH/PMTCT services at all levels
3. Provide integrated family planning services to HIV positive women and protect unwanted pregnancy
4. Strengthen continuous availability of good quality medicines, diagnostics and other essential supplies and commodities for PMTCT/MNCH
5. Strengthen leadership, management and partnership for e-MTCT of HIV programme at national, regional, zones and woreda levels to deliver effective and efficient services
6. Strengthen the Monitoring and Evaluation framework for e-MTCT of HIV and design strategies

Source: This table replicates the contents of a photograph taken of a banner on display at the Ministry of Health.
Note: MTCT is Mother to Child Transmission, FP is Family Planning, HAART is Highly Active Antiretroviral Therapy, ARV is Antiretroviral, MNCH is Maternal, Newborn, and Child Health, and PMTCT is Prevention of Mother-To-Child Transmission.

A discussion with team members at a rural health center, who did not offer their names, produced significant insight about health services provided by the government, along with a perspective on the role of religion. The material that follows came from respective interviewees and is combined in a way that provides the greatest clarity.[10]

According to these workers, religious attitudes in society do not ordinarily affect health-seeking behavior, but occasionally they do. For example, people regularly use the family-planning service and church elders support deliveries at the health centers. Elders of the church receive health training—a point emphasized by the rural health care interviewees. They then come back to their village and teach. This is the best way to get the health message to the community. For example, patients should continue to take prescribed mediation after they leave the health center and are more likely to do so if encouraged by elders.

"*Garee*" is the name for a group of about 30 women that holds scheduled meetings to discuss health-related issues.[11] The *garee* identifies potential solutions to problems. Health station workers and people in a *garee* have relationships with each other. Discussions move up from a *garee* to a level above—and then maybe up to the health center. The system, which started two years ago, is "well organized" but became fully operational only in the past year.

The town served by the health center encompasses over 150 *garee*, with a rate of representation at approximately one to five. These *garee* leaders in the community receive training at the health center. (Leaders are given "refresher training" by the rural health center as well.) Sub-teams from a given *garee* combine their plans upward to the *garee* level with help from extension workers. Used also for agriculture and education, the *garee* approach represents a "public mobilization" as encouraged by the national government.

Various positive results are reported at the rural health center in tandem with movement up from "a grass-roots level." Latrine coverage in town is 93%. Drugs are sufficient in quantity and there is a revolving fund for restocking. In spite of such positive results, some challenges remain: the rural health center lacks ambulances to transport pregnant

---

[10] Ten health extension workers, trained as nurses, are employed by the health center. Each worker receives about three-and-a-half years of training and can obtain a master's degree based on experience if they make the quota for admission.

[11] The *garee*, a secular rather than religious-based entity, is an institution not without controversy. Critics have claimed that *garee*-imposed actions, including punishments, can be implemented without due process. The *garee* system is identified with the ruling Oromo Peoples' Democratic Organization government (Tronvoll and Hagmann 2011: 199).

and high-risk women to a hospital. One interviewee reaffirmed that the town government provides vehicles for transporting high-risk pregnant mothers but requires reimbursement for gas. All chip in to offset the costs of transportation and there have been no deaths yet of mothers due to the ambulance shortage. More training for health workers would be desirable; nurses, specifically, are not given refreshment training. More professional development and continuing education would also be welcome.

What emerges from contact with the rural health center is an improving situation vis-a-vis the government provision of public health. Progress is limited, however, because of resources and reluctance among people to "buy in" completely when it comes to modern health care.

Religious entities, as pointed out by an official with the Ethiopian Catholic Secretariat, have provided health services for a very long time. The 1890s is identified by the official as the starting point among religious organizations for the provision of public health services in Ethiopia. An official with the Ethiopian Evangelical Church observes that it began in 1898 and offered health-related services from the beginning. An official from the Ethiopian Kalehiwat Church adds that "mainline churches have a long history," notably, in managing hospitals, and "people like churches providing services." This interviewee offers further observations about the work of churches in the health sector. The 12 clinics built by the Ethiopian Kalehiwat Church have focused on HIV prevention. Mennonites have also been active, through both clinics and schools. The "communist revolution," however, resulted in the nationalization of hospitals because the Dergue regime "saw churches as anti-socialist." Churches even closed down in some cases, especially in rural areas, and Ethiopia lost their development work as a result. With the drought-induced famine of 1984, however, a policy change ensued; out of perceived necessity, the Dergue brought churches back into development. The official from the Ethiopian Evangelical Church adds that most health activities in Ethiopia are currently carried out by churches.

The official from the Ethiopian Orthodox Church provides an overview of the institution's development. The Ethiopian Orthodox Church has 55 million members and belongs to the Consortium of Christian Relief and Development Associations. The Ethiopian Orthodox Church provides social services for people with HIV/AIDS. Health-related activities are "not a theological wing of the church." The official presented a comprehensive PowerPoint presentation on church governance and activities, including those in the health sector. This official emphasized that the 1974 revolution caused the church to suffer under decades of a Marxist/Leninist regime. As a result of that experience in particular, the Ethiopian Orthodox Church is working to minimize conflict. This point about church-related efforts toward cooperation is verified for Faith-Based Organizations in general by one of the professors from Addis Ababa University.

Three services, as summarized by one of the officials, are provided by the Ethiopian Evangelical Church to the public: (1) evangelism; (2) education; and (3) health. The Ethiopian Evangelical Church is "mandated to proclaim the Gospel" and "serve humanity," so the preceding wide range of services makes good sense. Since 1972, the official observes, the church has come up with ideas for ministry through community. This results from the interpretation of the biblical verse Mark 6—Jesus said "give them something to eat"—which has been interpreted as endorsing a "holistic" approach. Thus, from the Ethiopian Evangelical Church's standpoint, although the spirit must be fed, physical needs must also be met. (The Ethiopian Evangelical Church's holistic conception of caring for people, the interviewee notes, has been brought to the attention of the Lutheran World Federation.) Religion and health interact with each other, so it becomes natural to ask "What are we doing and why?" "Love of Christ" is the basic reason cited by the official for the Ethiopian Evangelical Church's attention to health. It is important, according to this representative, to sit with patients and listen to "how they feel."

Another official from the Ethiopian Evangelical Church reinforces the preceding points. The "vision of the church" includes a gospel wing and a development wing. The Ethiopian Evangelical Church's "livelihood development program" includes a wide range of considerations: food security, climate change, HIV prevention, education, youth health, protection of children from going onto the street, and concern for people living with a range of disabilities.

A doctor affiliated with the Ethiopian Evangelical Church draws attention to its role as a "pioneer" against health problems. Over the course of a century, work has expanded to remote areas, with significant Ethiopian Evangelical Church contributions to the MDGs and national development goals. According to one of its officials, the Ethiopian Evangelical Church has played a "vital role" in fighting HIV/ AIDS since 1988. A wide range of health challenges, such as malaria and communicable diseases, have been targeted by the Ethiopian Evangelical Church. At one point, the Ethiopian Evangelical Church had 59 health institutions, mostly in the west and south. However, as a result of shrinking financial support from abroad, the Ethiopian Evangelical Church now supports only about a dozen clinics, which are cheaper to operate. Seven or eight of the former Ethiopian Evangelical Church hospitals are now run by the government because financial support from abroad has been decreasing. Ethiopian Evangelical Church members, adds Negeri, are contributing money to replace the lost support from outside the country.

One official from the Ethiopian Evangelical Church sees churches and NGOs coming together to "help the livelihood of the needy." For example, 30,000 children without parents are being fostered by church programs. An example of a cooperative effort with other churches is "Act Alliance"; local and international churches have come together in a forum to share experiences and resources. The Consortium of Christian Relief and Development Associations is a rallying point for churches and other NGOs to: (1) discuss challenges and successes; and (2) aim for mutual learning.

Combating HIV through an inter-faith approach is a high priority for the Ethiopian Orthodox Church. One of its officials adds that the Ethiopian Orthodox Church has declared "war" on HIV/AIDS. While the subject is "difficult to talk about," the Ethiopian Evangelical Church pursues an ambitious approach that includes education, counseling, caring for those with HIV/AIDS, and assistance to orphans. The representative emphasizes that the public appreciates substantive results from efforts by the Ethiopian Evangelical Church in these areas. This official identifies other programs under the administration of the Ethiopian Evangelical Church. For example, "Water, Sanitation and Health," referring to the provision of potable water and the education of the public on hygiene (ie water and sanitary hygiene equal the "Wash, Sanitation and Hygiene" program), is a priority for the Ethiopian Evangelical Church. In sum, according to the church official, "integrated action" is contributing to improved health, along with the MDGs and the national development plan.

Ethiopian Kalehiwat Church provision of health care, according to one of its officials, is popular. This interviewee observes that the Ethiopian Kalehiwat Church has three health centers; other facilities have been given to the Ministry of Health. A professor affiliated with the Ethiopian Kalehiwat Church asserts that "we must work through religious organizations" to address public health. For example, this interviewee cites infant mortality as reduced because of efforts from religious entities.

A church official sees Catholic provision of health services as the simultaneous "promotion of evangelism and integrated human development." Coverage, as described by this interviewee, consists of 85 institutions that provide health services to communities, notably, in remote areas. General hospitals exist, along with more than 66 clinics and other facilities. There are 12 general health centers, four centers for orphans, 18 hospice centers for the dying and destitute, and about 2,500 health-care workers consisting of doctors, nurses, and technicians. In 2013, for example, the Ethiopian Catholic Church provided services to 3.5 million people. A specific priority is to reduce child mortality. Community-based health programs include various other projects: working with the Global Fund on HIV, involvement with more than 300 schools, the "Water, Sanitation and Hygiene" and "Peace and Justice" programs, and so on.

"Struggling with a high burden of infectious diseases," the Catholic official reports, is a preoccupation for Catholic health services. Other challenges persist. For example, the transportation of pregnant mothers to health institutions is difficult and causes a preference for delivering at home and the use of traditional midwifes. A waiting center is available for mothers with high-risk pregnancies. Women will tend to combine a visit to a health center with other activities, such as shopping. The Ethiopian Catholic Church has an "extension program" going house-to-house to encourage use of the health center. The goal is for each worker to reach 500 households in a six-month period.

Discussions with the Catholic leadership emphasized health education. Most notably, the "TeamStar" program has been operating for 14 years; its objective is to help students with a spiritual life to find their way regarding sexuality and fertility. The program operates for eight months of the year and reaches approximately 35,000 students and 70,000 parents. The program's focus is not on the Catholic value of abstinence. Instead, an official with the Ethiopian Catholic Secretariat observes that the church is trying to "figure out what is best" for young people. This interviewee added that TeamStar's efforts are linked to health posts, which benefit from church-sponsored efforts to promote health knowledge and awareness.

Services provided by the Catholic faith, observes an interviewee affiliated with that church, are in development work. The church is working on "values and mission" and provides services for all. The Catholic official noted earlier follows up with the hospice center as an example: there is "no preaching and people seek it out." People are referred there by government hospitals; they visit and then "feel good." This interviewee returns to the point that the church does not engage in religious activity in the hospice center. People "want their religious freedom," as the church official observes; they go to the church for service by committed religious Sisters, doctors, and nurses who are "not preaching." In sum, asserts the interviewee, demand is high because greatly needed services are conveyed without an evangelizing element.

Interviewees affiliated with the Ethiopian Catholic Church combine to emphasize the "holistic concept" in action. The specific illustration of this Ethiopian Catholic Church priority is the practice of home visits by Sisters. The Sisters are trusted and thus home vaccinations from them are more likely to be accepted. Accompanied by food, visits that entail vaccination exemplify a holistic approach to the treatment of body and mind.

An official with World Vision notes that the organization has had an official presence in Ethiopia since 1975. The organization possesses great experience in health care, especially with regard to nutrition and HIV. World Vision takes a comprehensive approach. Immunization is a long-standing priority of World Vision; further key concerns are food/agricultural security and child protection. World Vision's wide range of activities also includes emergency health programs for regions hit by disasters.

Provided by one of its officials, World Vision Ethiopia's (2013) *Annual Report* includes extensive information on the provision of health care by the organization. World Vision states its motivation for such efforts: "Our work is guide by our core values: Christianity, commitment to the poor, responsiveness, valuing people, partnership, and stewardship."[12] The report's section on "Health, Nutrition, and HIV/AIDS" (World Vision Ethiopia 2013: 12) asserts that World Vision has a new focus on "health system strengthening to contribute to the Ministry of Health efforts on reduction of maternal and child mortality." These activities include constructing and furnishing four new health centers, along with 23 health posts, and renovating 11 health facilities. World Vision has also targeted community members for training on maternal and childcare practices. HIV prevention training and support is a major stated emphasis as well. Another section of the report (World Vision Ethiopia 2013: 13) emphasized its efforts on water, sanitation, and health. Actions included the provision of clean water through wells, the construction of latrines at schools, and training in personal hygiene. In sum, the report communicated extensive efforts toward improved health care.

The Consortium of Christian Relief and Development Associations, as a Christian umbrella organization, includes a wide range of members. Religious entities are prominent within its ranks. Moreover, these Faith-Based Organizations exhibit "good structure from national

---

[12] www.crin.org/en/library/organisations/world-vision-ethiopia

to local levels." One participant in the group meeting observed that religious organizations are "active in the health sector"; their services include spiritual as well as treatment aspects. Faith-Based Organizations, for that reason, "are closer to community than government." Religious entities are "able to integrate their work with health care" and operate as "strategic partners" within the Consortium of Christian Relief and Development Associations. Furthermore, as described by another participant at the Consortium of Christian Relief and Development Associations meeting, religious partners reach out to communities in various health-improving ways. One point of emphasis is contacting new mothers a week or so after birth. A related ongoing project on polio asks mothers about immunization and provides "polio zero" to children.

As described by the Consortium of Christian Relief and Development Associations' members, development efforts are expansive and include water supply and health education, along with HIV prevention. Refugees are assisted in consultation with the UN. Various churches also coordinate on how to divide their efforts in border regions and meet with groups on the other side of the border "to compare notes." Cooperation occurs, for example, in the Gambela Region. When people are not willing to go to the Expanded Program on Immunization of the World Health Organization, religious leaders have helped with obtaining compliance. Expanded Program on Immunization coverage went from 15% to 72% because of the efforts of religious leaders.

What about the government in connection with Faith-Inspired Institutions with regard to the health sector? A World Vision official sees things "coordinating very well" at both federal and district levels. A positive working relationship exists; World Vision helps with capacity-building and is linked to the Ministry of Health. In the context of the Ethiopian Evangelical Church, a representative emphasizes a good relationship with the Ministry of Health. Government-based health facilities are "overcrowded," so faith-based facilities are more than welcome and used significantly. The opinion offered from the Ethiopian Catholic Church on this subject is also positive: "Thanks to the government," the interviewee claims, "we can create more health services." Government, this church representative observes, is able to help with developing health centers toward "blanket coverage."

An official with the HIV/AIDS Prevention and Control Office offers a positive view from the government side. This interviewee cites cooperative efforts against HIV/AIDS. Antiretroviral clinics, such as the one established in Soddo, include educational and teaching activities, along with counseling. There is also a hospital, St Peter, near the clinic. The government official notes that religious organizations, with the "umbrella organization" of the Ethiopian Interfaith Forum for Development Dialogue as a prime example, facilitate antiretroviral treatment and are highly active. Through teaching that reduces the stigma associated with HIV/AIDS, religious entities play a valuable role. This interviewee cites the specific example of a Catholic-based charity, St Luke, Missionary of Charity, which helps HIV-positive children.

Another official from the HIV/AIDS Prevention and Control Office also sees effective cooperation in place. An appropriate role, according to this interviewee, is played by religious leaders in a team effort against sexually transmitted diseases. People listen to religious leaders, so they are able to advocate effectively against harmful practices leading to HIV. This is how to "mobilize" a community. Clinics and health centers, in addition, are owned by religious entities. The government reacts very positively to efforts by the religious community regarding HIV in particular. Religious communities' contributions include stigma reduction, care, and prevention.

One official from the HIV/AIDS Prevention and Control Office is pleased that religious leaders have gained an understanding of HIV. The other official adds that the Ethiopian Orthodox Church has an HIV program. Some academic institutions, such as Johns Hopkins University, have been offering assistance. There even exists an organization of HIV-positive leaders: ETNERALE. One of the HIV/AIDS Prevention and Control Office interviewees notes that Faith-Based Organizations have become key partners who can help with education and advocacy. For example, the Patriarch of the Ethiopian Orthodox Church told people to "take the medicine with holy water" (ie "medicine" meaning antiretroviral drugs). With regard to HIV/AIDS, belief is increasing that the infected are "the same as others in the eyes of God."

The government official just noted, however, adds a point of caution: we must understand the "territories" of Faith-Based Organizations. For instance, these organizations cannot teach the use of condoms in a positive way. "Adultery," according to faith-based entities, "is adultery." It is reasonable to anticipate limits to the role that can be played by Faith-Inspired Institutions in support of implementation for modern medicine.

Opinions vary on the subject of government standards, which had changed shortly before the time of the interviews—a subject that came up throughout the discussions. Is it possible that the government set a high bar so it could take over religious hospitals? When asked that question, an official from the Ethiopian Kalehiwat Church argued that the government should have considered the full implications of its high standards prior to implementation. Private clinics are closing down because they cannot meet government standards—it is just too expensive to operate under the new rules. In addition, according to the interviewee, government standards are "complicated." Money for Ethiopian Kalehiwat Church health provision had come from the US President's Emergency Plan for AIDS Relief (PEPFAR), USAID, the Canadian Institute for Development Assistance, and other donors specifically for HIV work. Church provision of services to complement what is offered by the government, however, must now be self-supporting because external support is limited.

The interviewee from the Ethiopian Kalehiwat Church asserts that the public did not like the "handover" of clinics to the government. Clinics either upgraded to health centers or closed down. The manner of health-care provision matters as well. "Real care comes from empathy," the official claims, and churches are linked to that idea. As an illustration, people will choose to live out their final days in a religious facility. The interviewee from the Ethiopian Kalehiwat Church is "sad" about the impact of government policy: "we are doing good, but getting closed down anyway." The government, this official argues, should instead support faith-based efforts.

Consider Zambia and Burkina Faso as positive examples of subsidies in action. These cases, from the Ethiopian Kalehiwat Church official's standpoint, show how to "bridge the gap" between government and faith-based entities. A representative from the Ethiopian Evangelical Church adds that running a hospital is "too difficult" as outside support declines; the government, after all, has the option of financially supporting a church hospital rather than taking it over. The government should think about helping religious organizations to run clinics in a "sustainable, cost-recovery mode." The Ethiopian Evangelical Church, offers one of its officials, is aiming to do this itself.

An interviewee from the Ethiopian Catholic Secretariat notes the existence of church-sponsored health posts, clinics, centers, and general hospitals. The Catholic Church has two hospitals in partnership with the government, which subsidizes these hospitals by 9%. Based on new government standards, some posts may turn into centers and some clinics may be upgraded to hospitals or downgraded to posts. "Some clinics need to upgrade to health centers," which the interviewee from the Secretariat acknowledges as a challenge for the church. Upgrading is very expensive for the church in terms of "infrastructure and human resources." No clinic, however, has shut down; instead, they go up to a center or down to a post. No more clinics will exist; these operations had status above posts and below centers. The church makes the decision over which way to go, up or down. The Ethiopian Catholic Church, according to one of its representatives, prefers to upgrade its facilities. Fortunately, in some cases, a clinic is already meeting the new standards of the government and just a change of labeling is needed. The fate of a given clinic in a remote area, where there is no prospect of a government-run center being established anytime soon, would seem especially uncertain. The transition to meeting new government standards in remote areas "is a struggle" and, as the representative from the Ethiopian Catholic Secretariat points out, "we don't have much experience yet."

With regard to the overall character of provision, it is impossible to miss the concept of *holism*; it pervades discussion. Tables 5.2a and 5.2b, reproduced from banners on display at the Consortium of Christian Relief and Development Associations, confirm this point strongly. The first of the tables is from the Ethiopian Catholic Church. Its Development Commission emphasizes "integrated human development." The second table, from the Ethiopian Civil Society Health Forum, shows the range of organizations—20, of various kinds—involved in a variety of programs that link health to development.

Table 5.2a: Ethiopian Catholic Church

Ethiopian Catholic Church Social and Development Commission The Development wing of the Ethiopian Catholic Secretariat
Works to achieve ECC's fundamental mission—promoting an Integral Human development through:
• Promoting Quality Education Through the Church's Schools • Providing Holistic Health Care Services Through Ethiopian Catholic Church's Health Institutions • Ensuring Food Security, Livelihood and Enhancing Disaster Risk Reduction • Striving to Alleviate Problems Related to and Lack of Access to Safe Water and Proper Sanitation Services • Awareness Raising on Migration and Advocacy for Internally Displaced People and Refugees • Works to Empower Women and the Protection of Vulnerable Children and the Elderly

Table 5.2b: Consortium of Christian Relief and Development Associations

Consortium of Christian Relief and Development Associations Ethiopian Civil Society Health Forum
Background:
• Ethiopian Civil Society Health Forum is one of the thematic forums operating under the auspices of Consortium of Christian Relief and Development Associations. The forum was established in February 2012 by 20 interested CSOs working in the nation's health sector to provide basic health services in a coordinated and sustainable manner. The forum was launched on February 4, 2013 by HE Dr. Keseteberhan Admassu, Minister of the Federal Ministry of Health. Currently, the number of the forum members has reached more than 120. The forum has nine part-time steering committee members who lead the forum, and one full-time coordinator and assistant who facilitate daily routines and the implementation of health-related development programs. The forum has helped to enhance the visibility of CSOs, their role, and contributions at both country and global levels within a short time frame.

Source: These tables replicate the contents of photographs taken of banners on display at the Consortium of Christian Relief and Development Associations.

One Consortium of Christian Relief and Development Associations meeting participant argues that churches "must be involved in the holistic development of society." Activities at the Consortium of Christian Relief and Development Associations participant's church include Sunday School for youth, but also anti-stigma and discrimination regarding HIV/AIDS. These examples combine to reveal the holistic concept in action. Consider also the Ethiopian Evangelical Church website, which contains the following statement: "We have a deep concern, not only for the spiritual needs of a person, but also for his/her physical needs. Our motto of service is 'Serving the Whole Person', better known as, Wholistic Ministry".[13]

One professor, specifically noting an academic context, also speaks in favor of a holistic approach. Social work, from their point of view, entails "biology, psychology, and the social." All of those aspects matter with respect to healing. The professor urges the "appropriate participation of religious leaders in social work" and affirms that "spirituality matters." This academic interviewee adds further that "I don't fall apart easily because of my spirituality. I have three students working on projects in which religion plays a role."

An official from the Ethiopian Evangelical Church argues that prayer has a central value when people get sick. Medical treatment is essential

---

[13] http://www.wycliffe.net/organizations?entity=EEC&continent=AFR&country=ET

but people also value prayer. The Ethiopian Evangelical Church seeks to advise and comfort people—an effort to "respond to the whole person"—further confirmation of the holistic point of view. The Ethiopian government, however, is promoting secularism; according to the church official, "schools, including medical schools, are secular these days." How, then, can the Ethiopian Evangelical Church be expected to bring religion in to respond to indivisible human needs? Within a hospital setting, the church needs to listen to clients so that it can contribute effectively to observations written up on a given case. Therefore, the role of a minister in a hospital is "very important" in treating the patient as a whole person. For that reason, the trend toward secularism is seen by this interviewee as undesirable.

From a Muslim representative at the Consortium of Christian Relief and Development Associations group meeting came the holistic observation that the Quran calls for "treatment *and* prayers." Books exist on Islamic medicine. In addition, "Islam directs its followers to go to those who have knowledge" and books have been prepared for Imams on science and faith so that they can speak in an informed way about family planning. An emphasis exists on training Imams that faith and medicine are not contradictory. People need and use both spiritual and medicinal approaches. Prayer readings are available through broadcasts, 24 hours per day, and can serve various purposes, including reaching the sick. Islam has clinics and there is a focus on the value of vaccinations in the context of Islam. Moreover, fatwas have been produced on health.[14] Teachings in the fatwas are for Imams. The Imams, in turn, pass along the health message, in both Arabic and the local language, through sermons and social gatherings.

An official from the Ethiopian Orthodox Church observes that "science is not apart from religion." This interviewee goes on to say that "life is all-encompassing" and the Church must participate in "all areas." From its beginnings in Ethiopia, the Ethiopian Orthodox Church "has taken care of people, including health care." For example, the church has established health centers and some dioceses have their own clinics. For justification of church-related health services, the church official points to a book written by Saint Cyril, the Patriarch of Alexandria (376–444), interpreted to mean that "God gave wisdom to the physicians." Therefore, the church has no conflict with "modern medicine"; corporeal problems should be treated by doctors. The

---

[14] This is true elsewhere and with favorable results; see Roudi-Fahimi (2004) on family planning in Egypt and Iran, along with Kaufmann and Feldbaum (2009) on polio vaccination in Nigeria.

church will urge such treatment. "Physicians must be respected" because their wisdom is provided by God. The holistic point of view expressed here is clear to see.

What can be said, after this review, about the religious role in health-care provision? There is certainly a long history of this type of activity in Ethiopia. The religious contribution is badly needed because of limited service from the government combined with ongoing poverty. Various Faith-Based Organizations, such as the Ethiopian Orthodox Church, Ethiopian Evangelical Church, Ethiopian Kalehiwat Church, Ethiopian Catholic Church, and World Vision, carry out an impressive range of health-related activities. The Consortium of Christian Relief and Development Associations provides a point of coordination for the efforts of faith-based and other civil society organizations when it comes to health care. In an overall sense, the provision of health services among religious entities exhibits a holistic character.

Health workers at Addis Ababa University School of Public Health confirm the existence of traditional healers in their area, with "five or six licensed." Traditional healers and birth attendants, however, are being used less and are diminishing in number. One worker at a rural health center even stated that women in town no longer used traditional birth attendants. Health extension workers are having an impact and therefore herbalists and traditional healers "need to be integrated and work with us." In the words of one health worker vis-a-vis traditional medicine, "we need to decrease side effects." Unfortunately, according to one of the health workers at a rural health center, traditional healers "do not want to work with health professionals and that is a great problem." Some degree of conflict is therefore seen to exist between the traditional and modern sectors regarding health services.

Religion and health-seeking behavior

Religious beliefs, as a World Vision official points out, significantly affect the quest for health care. Consider this question, raised by a participant at the Consortium of Christian Relief and Development Associations group meeting: "Why would a religious person use contraceptives?" People are obviously affected by their religious background, with "lots of resistance even among the educated regarding behavior and attitudes." Faith-Inspired Institutions can be "very important for increasing demand," with a key role in "stigma reduction," along with advocacy, lobbying, and campaigning for health. All of the preceding items represent major contributions from religion that impact upon health-seeking behavior.

Religion is intertwined with resources in the explanation for the persistence of traditional healing as a choice among Ethiopians. "Health seeking is poor," observes an interviewee from the Ethiopian Catholic Secretariat, because it is not a priority for those with limited resources. It is important, especially in remote areas, to keep costs down. The Catholic official emphasizes limitations regarding mental health in particular. Health centers in rural areas lack resources, especially psychiatrists, to deal with mental health problems. Usually, only general hospitals have psychiatrists; sadly, people fear the mentally ill, which, in turn, worsens their condition. Mental illness has also been an issue for Ethiopians deported from countries in the Middle East. Refugee centers provide some "health, social, and integrative services" for Sudanese, Nigerians, and Yemenis. Overall, however, resources for mental health are scarce, which, in turn, encourages health-seeking behavior in the direction of traditional healing.

A professor from the School of Public Health, Addis Ababa University, draws attention to the importance of holy water in health-seeking behavior. During their experience as a nurse, a sick patient would request to leave the hospital to receive holy water. The interviewee said that she used to say "yes" because, if not, the patient would leave and likely never return to the hospital. The professor concealed those conversations from the attending physician. In addition, a sick person will have a "lottery" of church saints that are placed in a container and randomly drawn. So, if St George's name, for example, is drawn, then the sick person goes to the spring for holy water associated with St George. The interviewee believes in miracles of healing and gave the example of the recovery of a friend who had been diagnosed with breast cancer. This friend, who had received holy water, was later found to be free of cancer and remains in remission a few years later.

An official with the HIV/AIDS Prevention and Control Office echoes the observations of the Addis Ababa University professor: sick people prefer "holy-water places." Currently, Pentecostals seek "spiritual healing" and some stay in holy-water places for months. Another professor notes that some will claim that faith and holy water *supersede* medicine. This interviewee sees "confusion" on the part of some believers when they take antiretroviral drugs and holy water; there is fear that the medicine is "messing up" the effectiveness of the holy water. Priests, however, tell followers that it is fine to do both. Fortunately, belief in a likely positive outcome from combining faith-based healing—holy water, in particular—with modern medicine is increasing.

The chosen order of treatment is revealing with respect to the role of religion. A question during a visit to the Ethiopian Evangelical Church about the order of treatment (ie clinic versus traditional healer) produced a decisive reply. One interviewee observes that people come to a clinic after "cultural means" of healing. People do listen to doctors, but only once they get to a clinic. A doctor affiliated with the Ethiopian Kalehiwat Church adds that a minister will recommend a doctor after prayer.

Traditional healing and/or witch doctors are options for many in rural areas in the absence of trained personnel. Depression is seen as evidence of evil spirits and thus a Catholic official points out that the Sisters—in an aside to modern medicine—are trained to detect depression. In addition, according to a World Vision official, residents reported in a study on malnutrition that poor health could be attributed to the evil eye. Examples of such traditional beliefs are legion among interviewees.

Health-seeking behavior reflects a general belief among Ethiopians in the holistic character of people. A professor at Addis Ababa University asserts that the religious and physical worlds are closely intertwined. Further observations from a medical doctor and a theologian reinforce each other in support of that position. Consider the remarks of each in turn.

The medical doctor notes the common belief that the spiritual and material worlds are intertwined. This doctor reports that people "flock to spring water," usually close to an Orthodox church, and some even stay for months. Deep-seated belief in unseen powers, called animism in the West, persists in Ethiopia. The physician quotes a biblical verse to illustrate the point. In Mark 2, people carry a paralyzed man to Jesus, who says "your sins are forgiven." This is taken by the interviewee as an example of the "holistic nature" of people—a common belief among Ethiopians.

The theologian regards the ideology of "health and wealth" as an ongoing influence in Ethiopia. The standard, quite holistic, point of view conveyed by this interviewee includes spiritualism *and* modern medicine. Modern medicine is a "gift from God." For the theologian, Ethiopians occupy a middle ground of spiritual and physical health: education is gradually increasing the percentage of people who see illness in scientific as well as spiritual terms. Thus, holism, if anything, is on the rise.

What can be said, overall, about religion and health-seeking behavior? Religion clearly matters and its importance is intensified by resource scarcity. Traditional healing, with a notable presence for holy water, is a significant aspect of everyday life. Religion impacts upon the order of treatment, and some persistent beliefs, especially those connected to the efficacy of witch doctors, are harmful. Health-seeking behavior, in an overall sense, exhibits a holistic character among Ethiopians.

Traditional and spiritual healing

Traditional beliefs are significant. In Addis Ababa, a largely Christian area, World Vision made available a program on modern health care. Yet, many people still seem to prefer traditional healers, especially in rural areas. Despite years of health-care messaging witnessed by a World Vision interviewee, Ethiopians continue to seek out traditional healers.

An official from World Vision observes that people from around Lake Abaya, east of the Guge Mountains within the Southern Nations, Nationalities, and Peoples' Region, prefer to go to a traditional healer even if they live close to a health center. People tend to use non-scientific names that exist for illnesses; in other words, it is obvious that they have heard such terms from traditional healers handed down over generations. In particular, it is discouraging to the World Vision interviewee that malnourished children are taken to traditional healers. This is confirmed through interviews and focus groups. Overall, the official is "surprised" at the persistence of traditional beliefs and behaviors after nine years of work at World Vision.

A representative of the Ethiopian Catholic Secretariat observes that the real causes of childhood illnesses are not understood among many Ethiopians. Vaccination, another interviewee notes, can be associated with side effects such as fever and then linked to evil spirits. A polio immunization scar, along with crying and fever, will be seen as an ominous sign. Tefera adds that, according to traditional beliefs, human shadows may harm a sick child, which can cause a family to stay away from a health center. Shadows, along with having more people around, are believed to have a bad effect on a baby. An official from the Ethiopian Catholic Secretariat observes that the isolation of an infant can be good to keep them away from infection, but, at the same time, it is bad to eschew treatment.

Religious beliefs affect health in other indirect but significant ways, as pointed out by a professor from the School of Public Health, Addis Ababa University. For example, the Oromo have a traditional *hamachisa* leader. The leader is designated via the family and well respected and even authoritative within the community. An expectant mother needs the *hamachisa*'s permission to go to a health center to give birth, and there can be shame in not following this traditional leader's instructions.

Mothers also need permission for the vaccination and treatment of the childhood illnesses that are common in such a dry climate. A mother will "honor and thank" the traditional leader for their blessing. This is true, for example, in the Christian-dominated Amhara region. The previously cited professor observes that the Amhara region has traditional religious leaders, the *tankuwe*, who may be akin to a witch doctor. The professor's mother visited such a doctor. The interviewee posed the question of cause and effect about illness to themselves, asking, for example, what are the factors affecting malnutrition? The interviewee answered by saying a dry climate—not evil spirits.

According to this same professor, religious leadership at the local level is responsible for spiritual as well as material well-being. The role can be positive in terms of limiting deviant behavior. For example, consider the problem of open urination and defecation, which occur even in Addis Ababa.[15] This misbehavior is especially common among men. However, if found to be doing this in a traditional leader's area, the latter will decide on and effectively implement a punishment. Examples of sanctions include forced labor on land and collecting water from distant areas. The professor mentions that, in one sense, this process may not be ethical, but it does help to discourage behavior that, from a health perspective, is harmful.

Holy water, according to a member of the Ethiopian Orthodox Church, is used for either washing or drinking. From youth, Ethiopians are taught how to use holy water. The Ethiopian Orthodox Church, as described by this interviewee, believes that holy water can help those disabled, lepers, the blind, and so on. The Ethiopian Orthodox Church "believes in miracles," for example, applying soil and water from holy places to the body is expected to have healing power. Consider the Epistle of James: the priest is using water to counteract sin. In the Old Testament, the church member recalls, we find the example of Namaan being washed to take away his leprosy. In addition, soil around holy places is believed to cure disease. Tefera adds that people are buried at a monastery with soil regarded as blessed.

Speaking from an academic point of view, another professor from Addis Ababa University draws attention to the possibility that healing may be psychological. By going to the spring for holy water, "you

---

[15] The professor provided a document entitled "Latrine use and cultural values in rural population." It contained research from Year II medical students, supervised by the professor in 2005/2006. The research study assessed the range of cultural values related to sanitation and the use of latrines.

think you will be better and you are."[16] The professor said that drinking a quantity of holy water may have medicinal value since, incidentally, it is also mineral water. Alternatively, if you have a blockage in your digestion, the water could back up and make you worse. This interviewee remained noncommittal on believing in miracles when queried at that point.

One participant at the Consortium of Christian Relief and Development Associations meeting added that the use of holy water can coexist with modern medicine. However, pernicious effects from excessive belief in holy water also occur. For example, vaccination is mandatory for delivery but lack of follow-up after going home is common. People sometimes believe that vaccination brings "evil spirits," so they will prefer holy water.

All of this leads naturally into a discussion of ritual and iconography. A second professor from Addis Ababa University notes that the specific positions of holy pictures can be important. For example, Saint Mary is supposed to be at the south end of a church. In the Ethiopian Orthodox Church, men and women have separate positions (ie sides in the church building). Another professor from Addis Ababa University adds that people will put a Bible under the pillow to protect a child when parents leave the room or the child is sick.

Some people, an official from the Ethiopian Catholic Secretariat observes, engage in ritualistic activities. For example, maladies such as measles can result in a "coffee ceremony", which is a coffee making and consuming ritual. Consider ritualism also in relation to epilepsy. The mother of an epileptic child may prefer a church visit to a health center. "Ritual activity" in church, from the point of view of the faithful, is used to "release evil spirits from the body."

A third professor from Addis Ababa University identifies the "True Cross" as another place that people go for healing. (This artifact is claimed to contain a piece of wood from Jesus' cross.) A person who is ill will kiss a cross and then be blessed by the priest, who, in turn, prays for them and puts holy water or oil on their place of injury. Someone may also be submerged in water; this represents purification against sin more than an illness.

Ash from incense, observes a member of the Ethiopian Orthodox Church, is regarded as holy. Holy oil is used in tandem with ash. A container of oil is composed of oils from different plants. The priest prays over each oil and then combines them together. The new combined oil is then prayed over. He would then apply this oil to a

---

[16] The placebo effect is so strong that every pharmacological test controls for it.

location of injury or pain. Oil, according to this interviewee, may also be placed in or on someone's ears, shoulders, or forehead.

A fourth professor from Addis Ababa University draws attention to the value of a holistic approach to treatment. "Integration" of traditional and medicinal techniques can help in a synergistic way, for example, with HIV/AIDS. In response to a question about a hypothetical individual with a severe headache, this professor initially described the following sequence and then elaborated on the basics: (1) a church visit will ensue; (2) then treatment with prayer and holy water; and (3) then traditional healers with herbs (eg the boiling of leaves). The interviewee continued with the more specific illustration of eucalyptus leaves, burning incense, and using ash.

Priests, according to this same professor, would *not* approve of a person visiting a traditional healer. However, the professor stresses the value of an "integrated approach," which could be summarized as follows: priest → traditional healer → clinic → priest. The interviewee elaborated on the likely treatment of a headache, with Table 5.3 conveying the two options identified. In each instance, the role of traditional healing is quite evident.

Table 5.3: Treatment options

Option 1: Patient goes to priest	1. Receives prayer and holy water. 2. May also receive ashes from incense. 3. May also drink holy water. 4. Go to clinic, get evaluated, and get treated. 5. Go back to priest and report outcome—"give testimony." 6. Priest later tells congregation of healing of patient.
Option 2: Patient goes to traditional healer	1. May be prescribed eucalyptus oil, which is good for headaches. 2. Employ home treatments. 3. May also tie a cloth around head.

Spiritual and traditional healing, to sum up, continue to be significant in Ethiopia. Some controversy exists, however, on whether these features of the health system are stable or in decline. Holy water is a key part of the story with regard to spiritualism and traditional healing. So, too, are rituals and iconography in relation to health. The overall perspective that emerges from the interviews is a holistic sense of health, with traditional beliefs and spiritualism as elements that exist alongside modern techniques.

Evaluation of the role of religion in public health

Health services, an official from the Ethiopian Catholic Secretariat points out, present a great challenge in all of Africa. An official from the Ministry of Health observes that "formal religious institutions and informal beliefs have positive as well as negative impacts on health." A representative of the Ethiopian Catholic Secretariat asserts further that "both harmful and good values" come out of cultural traditions linked to religion. With these observations in mind, discussion now turns to: (1) the positive and negative roles attributed to religion; and (2) the virtually uniform criticism of the current role played by traditional healing.

Religious beliefs in general, as noted by an official from the Ministry of Health, can assist with health care. For example, religious leaders helped to get HIV rates down through a combination of moral and science-based teaching that, in turn, reduced the amount of risk-taking behavior. A representative of the Ethiopian Evangelical Church further emphasizes the need to educate people about "harmful traditional practices," which include female genital mutilation and early marriage (ie in relation to the psychological level of maturity). Pastors can and do tell congregations to wait for marriage and send girls to school instead, so religion can play a positive role in counteracting pernicious effects from traditional beliefs.

Religious leaders, according to the aforementioned Ministry of Health official, can play a valuable role in encouraging the use of modern medicine. These leaders are crucial in "social mobilization" and can teach their followers about positive health practices. Followers may even need the approval of religious leaders to obtain treatment via modern medicine. Eight to nine years ago, to cite a specific example, the Patriarch of the Ethiopian Orthodox Church took a leadership role in health. He openly told his followers at a holy-water site that "drugs and holy water are not antagonists." The net result turned out to be a great improvement in the lives of those who experienced being patients in the modern medical system. Thus, religious leaders can create awareness of scientifically based health care. In some instances, however, leaders still need to be convinced to play that role. Various religious organizations have their own health facilities—the Ethiopian Orthodox Church, Ethiopian Catholic Church, Seventh Day Adventists Word of Life, and others—that provide effective health care. This is invaluable because many people would not receive modern health care otherwise.

A representative from the Ethiopian Kalehiwat Church asserts that the institution is showing particular awareness of the value of seeing doctors. The Ethiopian Kalehiwat Church, for instance, is a "forerunner" in urging the acceptance of HIV as an illness, not a curse. About 90% of Ethiopian Kalehiwat Churches have an HIV-awareness department. Significant change in the acceptance of HIV is occurring as a result, and religious leaders and people of faith in the health sector are playing a key role. For example, the Ethiopian Christian Medical Doctors Association has helped with awareness. Nurses and doctors have worked to educate churches; as a result, hostile beliefs have eroded over a five-year period and larger churches responded to the initiative by setting up HIV departments. According to an official from the Ethiopian Kalehiwat Church, churches should feel responsible for taking care of people rather than blaming them and that mindset eventually took hold with regard to HIV/AIDS.

Interviewees identified a number of specific negative side effects regarding religion and health. A sample of their observations follows here:

- One Consortium of Christian Relief and Development Associations meeting participant emphasized harmful effects for treating illness through prayer unaccompanied by medical treatment.
- A professor asserts that people may stay too long at a spring for healing and also suffer from relying exclusively on holy water.
- Religion, according to another professor, can affect the health of a mother and child adversely. The *tankwe* or *hamachisa* must be given the first harvest of milk and even part of the first harvest from the field by the new mother.

Some experts focus in greater detail on negative aspects of religion in relation to hygiene in particular. A professor notes that, due to taboos, schistosomiasis is more common in Muslims. Hand washing is required for prayer five times per day, and since schistosomiasis is a waterborne illness, this can sometimes result in harmful effects. Some Orthodox churches, observes one professor, do not have latrines. This academic goes on to say that both Christians and Muslims can have improper bathroom habits because of: (1) a lack of education; (2) gender, that is, male dominance; (3) a lack of mixed bathrooms (ie the problem with using the same latrine is that the evil is in the toilet and may contaminate the spouse); and (4) poverty. Among the preceding reasons, the professor identifies (1) through (3) as "key," with (4) as a background condition.

Despite religion sometimes having positive effects on health care, the interviewees' assessments of traditional and spiritual healing, per se, went in a virtually uniform negative direction. Prayer, according to a doctor from the Ministry of Health, is not a substitute for treatment and "traditional beliefs lead to services that are harmful." The doctor focuses on a specific example regarding an injury. Consider a fractured tibia. A person with this injury may go to a traditional healer, but due to a tight stick attachment as treatment, the patient can end up with gangrene and amputation. Instead, they really need splinting from a doctor. This is *not* the same as the tight attachment of a wooden stick. What about, the physician asks as another example, a child who may appear at risk of polio? Assume that the child has acute paralysis of a limb. Under those conditions, a traditional healer should send the child immediately to a health facility. Traditional healers, however, are not good at referrals. They provide services beyond their knowledge to patients. "Traditional bone setters" in particular, the specialists in setting breaks, are often not competent.

Along similar lines, a member of the Ethiopian Evangelical Church asserts that those who initially saw traditionalists frequently come to a modern medical facility with "complications" from prior incompetent treatment. Use of traditional healers persists, but some people do seem to be learning from experience.

The doctor from the Ministry of Health is forthright about traditional healing, which is described as mostly "negative." For example, in the south-west of Ethiopia (Gambela Region), after birth, women cannot have intercourse with their husband for three years. This restriction regrettably produces marital infidelity as a by-product. (It is typical for a woman passing by such a home to simply come in and have relations with the husband.) More bad examples from traditional healing include: (1) applying dung on freshly cut umbilical cord; (2) giving butter to a newly born infant; (3) the extraction of infant teeth; (4) uvulectomy of a toddler so the throat is not blocked; and (5) female genital mutilation (especially in Afar and Somali—the two regions with the most extreme levels of cutting). All of the preceding practices reflect traditional beliefs.

An official from the Ethiopian Evangelical Church proffers the unfortunate case of a mother with her sick daughter. The daughter had been taken to a hospital for treatment of a "mental problem." Hospital treatment included instructions to get an X-ray. The X-ray produced a recommendation for treatment. Medical treatment via the hospital, however, did not produce improvement. Symptoms then became interpreted as "possession by spirits"; the mother, in turn, wanted holy water sprinkled. The holy water seemed to be successful, but the daughter soon became ill again. The mother took her daughter home to their location. The key point that emerges from this case is that people sometimes revert to traditionalism after modern medicine either fails or appears to have done so.

Latrines, especially in Amhara society, are associated with evil. While 95% of homes are estimated to have a latrine, one interviewee's study of usage suggests an actual rate of about 60%. Latrines, this professor observes, are linked in traditional beliefs to the presence of snakes and possibly even pythons. Small children are assumed to be innocent until the age of five and are not allowed to go near a latrine, the proximity to which is believed to make them sinful. Unfortunately, not using a latrine can spread diseases and make children ill or even cause death. The professor adds in a Muslim context that the door of a latrine must not face toward Mecca.[17]

Tooth extraction, as explained by the aforementioned professor, is one of the most common among harmful practices based on traditional beliefs. This is done to infants under one year old. Tattooing and uvulectomy may happen as well.[18] The first milk teeth are assumed to be bad and therefore removed by a traditional healer. Uvulectomy can also be a dangerous procedure because any existing infection can get worse. Another common practice linked to traditional beliefs is "vein cutting." This occurs when someone is sick with meningitis during the dry season. Vein cutting is intended to draw blood to presumably ease illness. This practice, of course, does not work and can make things worse.

Finally, witch doctors came in for universal criticism. One professor observes that witch doctors are private—not legal. They are criminals: "Smart guys make money cheating people." The professor adds that educated people do not go to witch doctors. Another professor notes that witch doctors are unacceptable to both Christianity and Islam. Visits to witch doctors, according to Kassaye, are secret and not socially acceptable.

Evaluation of the role played by religion in health care produces mixed results. Both positive and negative aspects are identified by interviewees. By contrast, criticism of traditional healing is close to universal. While a holistic perspective is taken by interviewees in an overall sense, they are emphatic about the need to temper devotion to the spiritual world with treatments from modern medicine.

---

[17] For an authoritative treatment of the issues in this domain, see Kumie and Year II Medical Students (2005/2006).

[18] The professor showed the research team scarification on his eyebrows where cuts are made to improve eyesight. The interviewee emphasized that this practice reflects traditional belief, *not* religion.

Processes and outcomes

Processes

Religion is of general importance in Ethiopia. Virtually all Ethiopians self-report as religious. Churches are widely seen as providers of guidance, notably, in important areas of life such as personal health. It is interesting to see how religious faith persisted despite the best efforts of the Marxist Dergue regime. One ongoing point of conflict concerns secular views associated with Western medicine as compared to the traditional beliefs held by many religious Ethiopians. This is a microcosm of tensions in Africa over secular versus religious beliefs.

With regard to health provision, religion plays an essential role. Religious organizations from abroad became active in health care back in the 1890s. Provision of health care reveals a religious cast in the sense that a widespread belief exists that physical and spiritual aspects of a person must be considered together in the context of treatment. This is certainly the position adopted by members of the Consortium of Christian Relief and Development Associations, a highly active umbrella organization of faith-inspired entities in Ethiopia. A point of criticism from the Consortium of Christian Relief and Development Associations' members, along with others, is that the raising of government standards caused some faith-based facilities to close. This unfortunate outcome tended to occur in the most impoverished areas, with no real replacement of even minimal services in sight.

Given those observations, this is a good point at which to pause and summarize the changes that took place in health care. The Health Extension Program started in 2004. This included the provision of salaries to Health Extension Workers, who are deployed throughout Ethiopia. The government can boast of some positive developments, even if gaps in quality and comprehensiveness still exist:

> [model households] go through an intensive vetting for graduation and are publicly recognized by local leaders after completing key health extensions practices at the household level. Model households also provide mentorship and act as role models for their neighbors. This has brought about impressive results concerning health outcomes resulting in significant reduction of harmful traditional practices, improved lifestyles and use of health services. (Damtew et al 2016)

Health-seeking behavior is greatly influenced by religion. Faith-based facilities are accessed regularly, at least in part, due to limitations in what the government provides. Moreover, the holistic sense of health—spiritual and physical elements taken together—underlies health-seeking behavior in general. This goes a long way in explaining preferences expressed for faith-based facilities, which are most open to the idea of a spiritual element in overall health.

Traditional and religious healing continue to play a significant role among Ethiopians. Traditional beliefs are expressed even among health professionals employed in the modern sector. Holy water plays a very important role in the holistic sense of health.[19] This is most prominent among Catholics but Coptics, for instance, also use holy water (Jacobsson 2002). The practice can be harmful, however, when it is seen as a substitute for modern medicine and inhibits or even prevents the proper treatment of illness.

What, then, is the overall evaluation of religion in the process of health care? Religion can and does play a positive role. A prominent example is with respect to health education, which is credited with reducing the HIV rate. Religious leaders also help in encouraging followers to access modern medicine. On the negative side, however, are harmful activities that take place when religiosity becomes extreme and traditional beliefs stand in the way of health-seeking behavior that is matched with illness. The state of health care will depend to a significant degree on building upon the positive and inhibiting the negative aspects of religious beliefs among Ethiopians.

Outcomes

Consider health care and outcomes, with special attention to women's health. Women in Ethiopia have had some problems that are similar to

---

[19] Traditional and religious healing plays a major role in efforts to treat mental health problems, along with psychosomatic disorders, throughout Ethiopia. Beliefs about these health challenges are relatively uniform among the major religions: "The differences between the main religions, Christianity in its two important versions, the Coptic and the Evangelical, and the Islamic religion are not so great in everyday life for many reasons. On the contrary, there is a great intermingling of these three important influences upon which modern scientific teaching and technology is superimposed through the schools and institutions which have been established in the country during recent decades.... This conformity in the basic philosophy of the different religious systems accounts for the fairly general view that severe mental disturbance is caused by evil spirits or evil supra-human beings possessing the mentally deranged or other evil forces like bewitchment and curses" (Jacobsson 2002).

their sisters in Uganda and Mozambique, but also some unique ones. As the Fistula Foundation (2017) reports (concerning the path-breaking fistula-treatment hospitals in Ethiopia), "Ethiopia is a country rich in culture and history but remains one of the poorest countries in the world." In addition, "the country's fertility rate is among the highest in the world, as are its maternal mortality and morbidity rates" (Fistula Foundation 2017). Additionally, Ethiopia has the second-largest refugee camp in the world, Dollo Ado, located along the Somali border, in the south-east (Fistula Foundation 2017).

Unfortunately, Ethiopia shows a gap between: (1) signing onto supranational or passing national mechanisms; and (2) their implementation. While it ratified the Convention on the Elimination of all Forms of Discrimination Against Women and "adopted it into its constitutional and legal codes," violations routinely occur (Make Every Woman Count 2016: 55–57). Many violations take place in the war-affected Ogaden region of the Somali Regional state due to the presence of the Ethiopian National Defence Force (ENDF) (Make Every Woman Count 2016: 55–57). Perpetrators in this group of rape, torture, and killings apparently enjoy immunity from prosecution (Make Every Woman Count 2016: 55). Government control makes media access and humanitarian assistance nearly impossible. Thus, there are no health services for rape victims in this region (Make Every Woman Count 2016: 56).

Consider the national level as well. While Ethiopia enacted provisions in its 2005 Criminal Code against female genital mutilation, domestic violence, extra-marital rape, and early marriage (including by abduction), many of these crimes persist (Make Every Woman Count 2016: 55–56). For example, the Mid-Term Review of the African Women's Decade cites a 2009 World Health Ogranization report that 70% of Ethiopian women reported suffering physical violence from their husband or partner. Rape as a tool of war persists into the present day; despite official penalties of five to 20 years in jail since 2005, it remains "one of the rampant crimes in Ethiopia" (Make Every Woman Count 2016: 56). Similarly, although Ethiopia passed a national law in 2001 raising the marriage age for women from 15 to 18, it is still reported that "as of 2015, one in five girls are married before the age of 18" (Make Every Woman Count 2016). In the Gondar region, almost half the girls under 18 are married. On a more positive note, there has been a decline in early marriage, from 30% to 20%, of girls who are 15–19 years old (Make Every Woman Count 2016: 56).

Ethiopia's (2014: 12) report on *Progress Toward Meeting the Millennium Development Goals* mentions the fact that it had endorsed those objectives and integrated them into its sectoral planning. The report highlights its internal and external coordination strategy for boosting the receipt of overseas development assistance from USD2 billion in 2001 to USD4 billion in 2013.

With regard to MDGs 2 and 3—access to primary and secondary education—the Ethiopia Country Report (Ethiopia 2014)[20] mentions the government's large investment in improving infrastructure at both primary and secondary levels from the mid-1990s into the 21st century. Based on its 1994 Education and Training Plan, Ethiopia has more than tripled the number of primary schools from 9,900 in 1994 to 32,048 in 2014 (Ethiopia 2014: 28–29). Comparable secondary school figures started at 346 schools in 1996, but rose up to 2,333 in 2014. In 1996, the national literacy rate reached 25%, but rose up to 47% by 2011 (Ethiopia 2014: 34). However, there is still a gap of 15 to 20 percentage points between the literacy rates of men and women nationally, showing that work remains to be done. As of 2015, 68% of women between the ages of 15 and 28 demonstrated literacy, as opposed to 41% of all women over 15 (Make Every Woman Count 2016: 56), and education matters so much in the context of health achievement.

With regard to MDGs 2 and 3—access to primary and secondary education—the Ethiopia Country Report (Ethiopia 2014)[21] mentions the government's large investment in improving infrastructure at both primary and secondary levels from the mid-1990s into the 21st century. Based on its 1994 Education and Training Plan, Ethiopia has more than tripled the number of primary schools from 9,900 in 1994 to 32,048 in 2014 (Ethiopia 2014: 28–29).Comparable secondary school figures started at 346 schools in 1996, but rose up to 2,333 in 2014. In 1996, the national literacy rate reached 25%, but rose up to 47% by 2011 (Ethiopia 2014: 34). However, there is still a gap of 15 to 20 percentage points between the literacy rates of men and women nationally, showing that work remains to be done. As of 2015, 68% of women between the ages of 15 and 28 demonstrated literacy, as opposed to 41% of all women over 15 (Make Every Woman Count 2016: 56), and education matters so much in the context of health achievement.

The Ethiopian government met MDG 4 of reducing child mortality by at least two thirds by 2014, likely one of the few African countries to have done so (Ethiopia 2014: 40). While its MDG 4 specific target

---

[20] www.et.undp.org/content/dam/ethiopia/docs/UNDP%20MDG%202014%20Final2Oct.pdf

[21] www.et.undp.org/content/dam/ethiopia/docs/UNDP%20MDG%202014%20Final2Oct.pdf

had been 63 deaths per 1,000 live births, Ethiopia reached its own internal metric of 60 in 2014. Perhaps not surprisingly, the report indicates that while infant mortality and that of children under five has been reduced in both urban and rural areas, the percentages outside of cities are harder to move (Ethiopia 2014: 43). Immunization rates have increased for childhood diseases covered in MDG 4, resulting in Ethiopia meeting the 90% target rate by 2014 (Ethiopia 2014: 45).

With regard to MDG 5a, the United Nations Economic Commission for Africa (2015) report states that Ethiopia (with the Congo and Nigeria in Africa) is one of six countries responsible for 50% of maternal deaths in the world. The country report states that while it has reduced maternal mortality from 1,400 deaths per 100,000 in 1990 to 420 in 2013, Ethiopia would not reach the 75% reduction goal of MDG 5a of 267 such deaths by 2015 (United Nations Economic Commission for Africa 2015: 47).

Similarly, Ethiopia is one of 21 country targets of the Global Plan to eliminate new HIV infections in children by the year 2015 (UNAIDS 2017). As the summary notes:

> in 2009 there were 270,000 new HIV infections among children in the 21 Global Plan priority countries, only 36% of pregnant women living with HIV had access to recommended antiretroviral medicines to prevent transmitting the virus, and just 15% of children living with HIV had access to life-saving anti-retroviral therapy. (UNAIDS 2017)

By 2011, seven of the 21 countries (including Uganda, at 86%, and Mozambique, at 75%) had reduced new HIV infections among children. By 2013, Ethiopia had reduced it by 50% (UNAIDS 2013). Still problematic, however, is the fact that as of 2015, "only 24% of pregnant women who are eligible [for HIV services] receive them, and 1/3 of children born to an HIV-positive mother is infected with the virus" (Make Every Woman Count 2016: 56–57).

With regard to MDG 5a, one doctor notes that the contraceptive prevalence rate in Ethiopia increased from 6% in 2004 to 40% in 2014—an enormous success (Mortada 2014). Due to a desire to meet MDG targets, the Ethiopian government obviously desires to push the contraception prevalence rate up and the illegal abortion rate down (PRI 2014; Provost 2014). In a country where 95% of the population is Muslim, Orthodox Christian, or evangelical Protestant, the national government performed a tightrope act in 2005 and decriminalized abortion in the cases of rape and incest, severe fetal defect, or "if the mother was under the age of 18 and could not care for the baby herself" (Mortada 2014). Prior to 2005, illegal abortions had been blamed as the number one contributor to maternal mortality (PRI 2014). Within three years of the 2005 decriminalization, 27% of women had legal access to abortions. The increase in the number of women having abortions legally resulted from a decision by the Ministry of Health not to require women to state their reason for access (Mortada 2014; PRI 2014).

Conflict persists among religious representatives over abortion in Ethiopia. On the one hand, a conservative Protestant group called Christian Workers Union for Health Care in Ethiopia publicly demonstrated against the government's liberalization in 2005 (PRI 2014). On the other hand, despite the noted social conservatism of Ethiopian society, some clergy and others have been interviewed as saying that they recognize that safe abortion is the lesser of two evils.[22]

Estimates for Ethiopia in 2009 suggest that "there was only one doctor for every 50,000 people" (Provost 2014). Moral and financial pressure on Ethiopia comes through the MDGs; "in pursuit of the MDG's, the Ethiopian government has remodeled its entire health system" (PRI 2014). Ethiopia's problems are a combination of: (1) being the second most populous country in Africa; and (2) having serious infrastructure and access issues. In 2003, the government implemented a Health Extension Program to train young women in preventive care and services, who then became placed in rural villages. This program increased in 2011 and became known as the "Women's Development Army." In addition, a "health army," comprised of thousands, works in tandem with "salaried, trained extension workers." The health army concept is based on 16 priority interventions related to the MDGs, such as vaccinating children, having separate latrines, sleeping under mosquito nets, and using birth control (Provost 2014).

Families who adopt most or all of the suggested 16 components become "model families," and receive certificates and public recognition in the village. These families are then asked to help work with others not yet reached by the program. Another positive part of this change through publicly identified agents is, for example, the targeting of "cultural and attitude-related bottlenecks" that can limit women's

---

[22] For example, a local priest in Mosebo is quoted as saying "children are a gift from God, but having more children than you can feed is an even bigger sin" (Mortada 2014). A health worker noted that while his religion forbade abortion, "for me as a human being I accept it is necessary" (Mortada 2014).

willingness to access comprehensive reproductive services. In particular, some women feared going to health facilities to deliver their babies since the stretchers used to carry them had been designated as "bad luck" in some views. The government response to that problem included changing the stretchers and incorporating elements of traditional ceremonies, including coffee, traditional food, and religious leaders, into the facilities at which the birth is taking place (Provost 2014).

Traditionalist beliefs, population density, conflict-ridden regions, and poverty have all combined to hurt girls and women in two specific ways. The first is that Ethiopia is one of the three countries in Africa with the highest rates of female genital mutilation, despite the 2004 law banning it. Figures state that as of 2011, 74% of women in Ethiopia had suffered from this (28tooMany 2013).

Another issue is related to child marriage: the problem of fistula. (This is true whether the marriage is a product of abduction or not.) Fistula occurs when a (usually) young woman labors too long and tearing occurs, creating an abnormal passageway either between two organs or an organ and the body's exterior. Women with fistulas are often shunned by their families, even requiring them to live in the bush. Unfortunately, the characteristic odor can also make them prey for animals (Hamlin Hospital 2017). Australian doctors Catherine and Reginald Hamlin opened the first and largest hospital in the world dedicated to the treatment of obstetric fistula in 1974. Since that time, they (and she since his death) have opened five more regional centers in Ethiopia. There are only 150 hospitals in Ethiopia and many rural women live several days' walk away from treatment centers, so the availability of regional centers is crucial.

Additionally, the Hamlins opened the Hamlin College of Midwives since, at one time, Ethiopia had only 7,000 trained midwives (and 250 practicing ob/gyns [obstetrics and gynaecology personnel]) for a population of over 90 million (Hamlin Hospital 2017). The childbearing population ratio between pregnant mothers and midwives is thus 1:14,000, nearly three times the World Health Organization-recommended figure of 1 midwife per 5,000 births (Hamlin Hospital 2017). Another hospital working in Ethiopia on this issue is the Aira Hospital, operating as a "nonprofit institution owned and administered by the Ethiopian Evangelical Church Mekane Yesus" (Hamlin Hospital 2017). This hospital serves an "estimated 40 to 50 thousand citizens per year" (Hamlin Hospital 2017). In 2014, the government created a five-year campaign to eliminate fistula and has committed many resources to this venture (Fistula Foundation 2017). Another outreach program of the Aira Hospital is to partner with Women and Health

Alliance International (WAHA) to provide such care at the world's second-largest refugee camp, Dollo Ado (Fistula Foundation 2017).

Overall, given large challenges from demographics, war, poverty, and traditional beliefs, Ethiopia has been quite slow to modernize its treatment of women. Some exceptions exist. Ethiopia's contraception prevalence rate, for instance, is roughly three times higher than Mozambique's, according to the World Health Organization (2015) report. The World Health Organization report tempers the claim by some Ethiopian doctors of a contraceptive prevalence rate of 40%, instead situating it at 29% (World Health Organization 2015: 89–96). In the same source, Uganda's rate is situated at 30% and Mozambique's at 12%.

With regard to MDG 6, the HIV/AIDS prevalence rate in 2000 already stood at the 2015 target (4.5%). It has been reduced to 1.1% by 2014, a rather astonishing decrease (Kafeero and Birungi 2014: 52). The story becomes less positive when we focus on rates for women, who show an infection rate twice that of men (2% versus 1%). Furthermore, women between the ages of 30 and 35, depending on region, have a prevalence rate between two and six times higher than that of men in the same age group (Kafeero and Birungi 2014: 53–55). As in Mozambique, HIV/AIDS in Ethiopia is much more often an urban than rural disease. The Ethiopia report mentions that the country has met its target of reducing HIV/AIDS among those in the 15–24 age group (but clearly not in those a decade older). In part, Ethiopia reached the younger group due to integrating HIV/AIDS treatment into "all its sectoral health plans" and by increasing the reach of its free antiretroviral services, including to mothers (Kafeero and Birungi 2014: 55–56).

Summary

Religion plays an essential role in Ethiopia with regard to both the provision and seeking of health care. Ethiopians convey a holistic view of health, in place for a very long time. Traditional healing continues to be important; even those who believe in modern medicine may begin their process of health-seeking with that option. Holy water is taken quite seriously in Ethiopia—perhaps, at times, posing a threat to health when modern techniques are neglected in favor of it. This point can be carried forward in a gender-related context because of the likely role of traditional thinking in holding back some outcomes for women, as revealed by a review of the MDGs. Overall progress is evident, however, with the role of religion in the provision and consumption of health care as a primarily positive part of the story.

6

What have we learned?

Overview

Religious belief plays an important and, for many, central role in the lives of people around the globe. This is especially true of Africans, and research from preceding chapters on Uganda, Mozambique, and Ethiopia is in line with that assertion. Religion provides meaning, relationships, and a world view. These beliefs, in turn, affect people's behavior in many domains of life. One important area relates to health care. When people are sick or injured, they seek medical assistance for the means to restore health. This is true for individuals with differing religious beliefs and for those who profess no particular religious belief. The meaning of medical assistance, however, can be more comprehensive—with an essential spiritual component—for people of faith.

This chapter unfolds in four additional sections. The first section covers processes of health-seeking behavior and provision in Uganda, Mozambique, and Ethiopia. Second, outcomes are reviewed for the three states. Third is a summing up of insights from the research in relation to processes and outcomes. Fourth and last comes theorizing that could stimulate future research. This takes the form of a conceptual model for religion and health care in Africa.

Processes

How do religious or non-religious beliefs affect how health care is both provided and understood? This book has examined the relationship between religion and health to understand better how they relate to one another. Three case studies have been drawn from Africa for a number of reasons. First, and as noted at the outset of Chapter 1, Africa has 13% of the world's population but 24% of its disease burden (Cooke 2009). Second, Africans are a very religious people; understanding how their beliefs interact with seeking health care provides important insights into obtaining more efficient, effective, and culturally sensitive ways of provision for Africa.

Answering the question of how religion is connected to health in Africa requires a response that may be summarized as define, measure, capture, and integrate. The first two challenges are those of definition and measurement: how best to define and develop ways to measure religious beliefs and behavior and the impact of these factors on the supply and demand of health care across such a vast and diverse continent. Another challenge—once the first two had been met—took a more practical form: how best to logistically gather data in Africa to address these design questions. A final challenge is how best to integrate the varied academic approaches of researchers who had backgrounds in health care, social science, non-governmental organizations (NGOs), religion, and medicine.

Results from the chapters on Uganda, Mozambique, and Ethiopia all confirm the impact of religious beliefs on health perceptions, procurement, and provision. The investigation also discovered substantial variation by country and encountered some surprises. It is universally held that good health is a key aspiration and that modern medicine is a means to that end. No matter the religious belief of the individual, all showed awareness of the importance and efficacy of medical treatment. Research from the three African countries revealed no significant differences among Christians, Muslims, and followers of traditional African religious customs in this respect.[1]

To yield useful results, the study further analyzed the relationship of health and religion by taking apart the pieces and seeing how they fit together. Two elements are evident in understanding the relationship of religion and health care in Africa. The first element relates to the provision or supply of health care. The second element concerns the demand for health care on the part of citizens in the country. The demand side relates most directly to the health-seeking behaviors of individuals who may or may not be sick. In this area, cultural factors such as religion affect what economists call "taste" in preference for services. The public health field describes these as health-seeking behaviors. The main point is that people are sick and want to get better, and they go about this in ways that they think will maximize that end given the constraints of time, money, and the beliefs they possess.

Further disassembly reveals that the supply of and demand for health care possesses both a structural component and a discernible process at work. For structure, the supply-side features include health-care

---

[1]   As acknowledged toward the outset of this study, the research is based solely on states with Christian majorities and a Muslim minority. Whether results would hold in a Muslim-majority state is a question that cannot be answered yet.

institutions and regulations. The supply of health care may be met on the ground through secular, Western, faith-based, or traditional methods. Ownership of these institutions may alternatively be through the state, such as the Ministry of Health, or NGOs. The three countries examined in this book all include examples, along with the limited data available, of medical care supplied by state-run hospitals or clinics, faith-based ones, or traditional methods of delivery. The regulatory framework varied from one country to the next, but all three countries accepted these very different types of delivery. Quality of care, which also differs among these three means of health-care conveyance, will be discussed later in this chapter.

Variations due to geography, income, and capacity also affect the supply of health care. The countries examined in this study are largely rural. Each country contains a typical, by developing world standards, prime city of several million inhabitants. This political and economic hub dominates the country. Nevertheless, and importantly, most citizens do not live in the capital. As a result, regulations and policies written in the capital city do not always get implemented outside of it. Even within rural areas, there is a marked difference in settlement patterns. Some rural areas are connected very well to transportation, electrical power, and communication links. These features greatly facilitate the supply of health care. Other rural areas have much less access to other parts of the country and the delivery of health care is impeded as a result. It is important to note that the demand for health care is not lower in these areas, but the ability of people to access it is quite limited. Health care is an unmet demand.

The procedural component of demand recognizes it as a moving target. It is not a static demand; rather, people, policies, politics, development, and preferences are constantly changing. For example, even though much of the population in the three countries studied is rural, there is a very large movement of people to the cities. This is particularly true for younger people, who are leaving the rural areas and moving to the cities in search of jobs and the amenities afforded by a larger urban area.

Urbanization—the process of moving from rural to urban areas—is but one aspect of this dynamism seen in Africa. Another dynamic at play in the delivery of health care is the changing regulatory process. Aspects include standards, licensing, and the provision of different types of medicine. For one example, HIV has posed a major health challenge to Africa for the past two decades. The regulatory environment shifted in response to foster the delivery of antiretrovirals, the setting up of means to ensure compliance with the drug regimen, and other methods of prevention. Another dynamic observed is the gradual extension of health care by the government into more rural areas. The cumulative effect of this incremental process has been to integrate the population into a comprehensive health-care delivery strategy. In Ethiopia, for example, the "*garees*" have been an important method by which the government has attempted to improve health care for the rural population. Finally, technological changes such as the cell phone and the Internet have enabled the delivery of health care to be more efficient.

The second element is the demand side of the equation. While it is in many ways self-evident that someone who is sick wants to get better, a number of factors influence how the goal is best achieved. The case studies of Uganda, Mozambique, and Ethiopia all illustrate how demand is influenced by the internal and sometimes competing effects of religious commitment and modernization, as well as by world views about the cause of illness. These factors influence health-seeking behaviors for people in the countries examined. In most cases, people avail themselves of both traditional and Western-style modern medicine. What is most interesting, and one of the main contributions of the study, is the understanding of how, why, and where people tried to get better. A dynamic on the demand side is fairly clear for all three countries. In the case of Ethiopia, there is rising demand for giving birth at clinics rather than at-home births. Increasing educational levels, particularly for women, are also leading to changes in health-care demand.

Besides the structural and procedural aspects of the health-care system, there is also a context that provides additional insight into how religion and health care relate to each other. In looking at the history of health-care provision for the three countries examined, all share a number of features. In each case, health care had traditionally been provided by local individuals trained in indigenous means and understandings of well-being. The word "traditional" means recognition of a more holistic approach to health care that includes both the physical nature of the illness and a possible spiritual connection. The population widely trusts and accepts traditional healers.

Christian missionaries began evangelizing the interior of Africa in the late 19th century and brought with them modern, Western means of health care as part of their evangelism efforts. For the Christian missionaries, not only was the improvement of one's spiritual condition vitally important, but so, too, was the enhancement of physical health and education. Missionaries therefore set up churches, clinics, and schools to improve the spiritual and material condition of people in what are now the independent countries of Ethiopia, Uganda, and Mozambique. The regulatory environment for medical care also changed with the subjugation of Africa under colonial rule after the Berlin conference in 1885. Although these health policies varied by colonial power, colony, and even district, they still fostered the supply of medical care in the three countries. Ethiopia is perhaps the most interesting case because it never really fell under colonial rule. Christian missionaries, nonetheless, began introducing Western means of medical care at approximately the same time as in Uganda and Mozambique. The government of Ethiopia, again, not under colonial control, also encouraged these efforts. The Dergue regime in Addis Ababa had a world view of secular socialism, which included a commitment to Western medicine, though its reach remained limited.

As a result, in Ethiopia, local methods of supplying health-care retained importance. Health care supplied by traditional healers included the physical isolation of sick patients to avoid the "shadow." Other medical procedures included cutting eyebrows or putting tattoos on the temple of the head to improve eyesight. This concept of the shadow points out concern expressed towards negative aspects of traditional healing, commonly called witchcraft. The Ethiopian Orthodox Church similarly supplied health care, though in ways markedly different than earlier, Western-based religious organizations with less of an emphasis on modern medicine. The church's major means of supplying health care included prayer, holy water, holy sites, the soil from holy sites where saints are buried, and holy oil.

As the colonial era progressed, the supply of health care began to take recognizable form. A triad emerged for health care supplied to Africans. First came care by traditional healers, which included a concern for the spiritual and physical condition of the patient but lacked access to treatment protocols and medications increasingly available in the West. This included many different traditional health-care services: curative, general traditional health care, mental health care, midwifery, bone setting, and so on.[2] Modes of administration for medications include "oral ingestion, steaming, sniffing of substances, cuts (the African traditional medicine form of injection) and/or body piercing (the African traditional medicine form of acupuncture)" (Mhame et al 2010). Even today, traditional healers arguably remain the most important means for many people to obtain health care. Second came health care through clinics and hospitals supported by religious organizations, largely Western in background, culture, and medicine.

---

[2] Detailed descriptions of these medical practices are available in Mhame et al (2010).

Government clinics or hospitals provided by the colonial authorities became the third type of supply.

These three means of supplying health care survived intact into the post-colonial era. In the cases of Ethiopia and Mozambique, the coming to power of secular, ideological, and Marxist governments led to the suppression of the supply of traditional and faith-based health care in favor of government-run facilities. In effect, health care became nationalized, or, more accurately, the government attempted to achieve that goal. The radical governments of these two countries, however, lacked the capacity to effectively implement their objectives on a national basis. Furthermore, while it proved relatively easy to take over the faith-based hospitals, respective governments could not nationalize "traditional" health care. This looked even more obvious as both Ethiopia and Mozambique became enmeshed in long-running and brutal civil wars. These wars damaged health-care infrastructure and also limited the ability of governments to provide such services. For many Ethiopians and Mozambicans, these developments essentially limited their options for health care to traditional healers.

Stagnating economies in Africa in the decades following independence, conflicts engendered through the Cold War, and lack of government capacity in all three countries led to increasing foreign involvement. Interventions in the provision of health care for citizens came from foreign countries, multilateral organizations such as the United Nations (UN), and NGOs. These governments and organizations provided increasing amounts of money and technical expertise to improve the delivery of health care in all three countries. The effective globalization of health care in Africa led to areas of marked disagreement between the donors and recipients of aid regarding certain issues and policies.

One of these policy areas observed in Chapters 3–5 relates to what is often called reproductive health. Although the meaning of this term is broad, one aspect of it is a right to an abortion. Another area highlighted, central to Millennium Development Goal (MDG) 5b as well, is contraception. Important in those preceding areas is that all three countries under study include a significant Roman Catholic population. The Roman Catholic Church, along with some others, cites theological reasons for not supporting the use of artificial birth control. In those cases, pragmatic solutions have been developed in the countries studied—particularly Uganda—to address religious concerns. Muslim and Protestant faith-based NGOs supply condoms and birth control pills to the population, including Roman Catholics. In some policy areas, such as female genital mutilation (FGM), by contrast, there is a growing consensus between donor and national health-care providers about the importance of ending the cultural practice.

Striking differences are observed among the three countries as to how elements of the health-care delivery triad relate to one another. These three approaches could be summarized as dispatch, deny, and develop. These three approaches may simply have reflected the religious realities on the ground given the varying degree of traditional beliefs recorded in each country, as seen in Table 2.1. In Ethiopia, the government and faith-based religious groups worked together, even if in a largely uncoordinated manner, to sideline traditional African health care. In Uganda, traditional health care existed as a very strong component in the country. Among many government and health-care leaders, an attitude of denial of its importance, however, remains relatively common. Many of these interviewees expressed the belief that traditional medicine had been important but would increasingly become irrelevant in a modernizing Uganda. This assertion may or may not be true, but it is clear that traditional means of health-care delivery remain important for many people in the country.

Mozambique's development of missionary hospitals and clinics historically stayed at a lower level than in the other two countries. Nationalization of faith-based hospitals and clinics by the Marxist government in the 1970s further reduced their importance. From a market viewpoint—although the then Marxist government might not see the irony in this statement—its policy essentially eliminated one important competitor for African traditional religion. The struggle for independence and the civil war further eroded what modest ability the new post-independence government retained to provide health care. As a result, traditional health care within Mozambique maintained the greatest observed level in any of the three countries. The response of the regime has been to recognize the importance of traditional healers and seek not to eliminate them, but to co-opt or incorporate them into a government-run health-care approach.

Another finding of the research in this volume is that a religious world view tends to see health in a broader manner than simply physical or material. One's health is also clearly related to the spiritual condition, though it is not always obvious how this plays out for any given individual. What differs markedly is the degree to which the physical, emotional, and psychological aspects of the individual remain separate from the spiritual. More traditional Christians (and, as far as one could ascertain, Muslims) believe that the physical body may be healed apart from an underlying spiritual cause. There may, however, be an epiphenomenal spiritual cause that would require prayer.

Newly emerging charismatic churches from the West—notably, Pentecostal—and traditional faith healers both see the physical, mental, and emotional spheres of an individual as being embedded within a larger spiritual sphere. Emerging churches and traditional healers thus focus on understanding spiritual causes to heal the individual. Although they hold very similar views of the relationship between the spiritual and physical world, this similar metaphysical world view nevertheless places them more in competition with one another. Charismatic churches would see any spiritual source from outside of God as a false belief and potentially witchcraft, which is forbidden. However, criticism laid at both groups by health professionals asserts that the healing is ineffective, is inappropriate, delays the intake of patients into a hospital, and is done for financial gain.

Government health ministries are all well aware of differing perceptions of health, medicine, and belief. The government (and other Christian groups, it might be added) had more conflict and differences of opinion with the emerging churches due to their size, sophistication, and power. In Mozambique, the government failed to co-opt emerging churches such as the Igreja Universal do Reino de Deus. In Uganda, the government health ministry supported the role of religious belief (though less enthusiastically so for traditional healers) and institutions in providing for the health of citizens. In fact, the government encouraged these efforts and also subsidized religious-based hospitals and clinics.

Research confirms the critical role of religious individuals and faith-based institutions in delivering health to citizens. In Uganda, for example, over half of the health care in the country is faith-based. Administrators at Muslim hospitals also mentioned how their institutions managed to meet the health needs of Ugandans. In Mozambique, a Mozambican Presbyterian official pointed out that during the colonial era, the Presbyterian Church operated a number of hospitals. The new Marxist government upon independence seized those facilities, the official added. Mozambicans working in health care for World Vision also mentioned the critical role of Christian NGOs in meeting the health-care needs of the population.

On the health provision side of the equation, there is some competition among religious groups. This is especially true between Christian churches and traditional healers on the nature of spiritual healing. Christians interviewed acknowledged that some traditional healers wished to do well, but that not all did. Serious theological differences also exist over the source of spiritual power. This matter seems to be less of a concern among Muslims, at least in Mozambique, who apparently had a greater disposition to be syncretistic. This is one area requiring additional research. Both Christians and non-Christians distinguished between traditional herbal medicine and spiritual actions. One Ugandan health official stated a willingness to take a traditional medicine for a headache but would not support "funny stuff" by traditional healers.

Overall, religious belief is important to individuals' world views and affects how they understand health-seeking behaviors. Clearly, there are other variables besides religion, such as education, income, rural/urban location, and distance from the nearest clinic, which influence health-seeking behavior and provision. Nevertheless, it is evident that the religious factor is one that needs further investigation in Uganda, Mozambique, Ethiopia, and beyond. The importance of religion offers strong confirmation of the Social Determinants of Health frame of reference that guides this research.

Outcomes

Observations are comparative and begin with a discussion of context. The assessment will zero in on demographic change and reproductive health. Analysis finishes up with a link to policy as influenced via multi-level, supranational mechanisms and alliances for change in health care.

Ethiopia and Uganda are in similar situations regarding recent wars and inter-ethnic strife, according to the Berlin Institute for Population and Development (2014). In a phase of recovery from strife, each state faces demographic challenges from rapid population growth. A comparative analysis of Ethiopia and Uganda conducted by the Berlin Institute, which draws attention to demographic nuances while affirming rapid population growth for both states, is reproduced in the Appendix (see p 198).[3] While both states are challenged by rapid change, Ethiopia has done much more than Uganda to promote contraception and public health, which impacts upon MDG 5b.

While the Ugandan system of health provision is insufficient (similar to Mozambique's) both for preventing pregnancy and dealing with the majority of high-risk pregnancies that are borne by young women, Ethiopia has put national and international money into its population plan. In both Ethiopia and Uganda, the population is predominantly rural (at 83% and 85%, respectively) (Berlin Institute for Population and Development 2014: 2). The rural population of Mozambique is a somewhat lower proportion of the total (at 68%) (TradingEconomics.

---

[3]   A comparable analysis is not available for Mozambique.

com no date). As reported by the Berlin Institute for Population and Development (2014: 2):

> The Ethiopian government invests more money in providing contraception than any other country in Sub-Saharan Africa. In 2010, public bodies in Ethiopia spent 15.9 million dollars on contraceptive procurement: 60 percent of these funds were provided by the State with the remaining 40 percent provided by international organisations. In contrast, the Ugandan government provided almost no support for family planning.

As with the two other countries, it is more difficult for rural women to access reproductive health care than those in urban areas. However, due to the Ethiopian government's investment, urban women report their increased use of modern (chemical) contraception, from 30% to 50% during 2000–2011. In rural areas, the increase has been more noticeable, from 3% in 2000 to 23% in 2011. Women in both areas report less-than-optimal access to hormonal injections, their preferred type of contraception (Berlin Institute for Population and Development 2014: 3). According to the Ethiopia Country Report, married women reported only an 8% contraceptive prevalence rate in 2000 as opposed to a 42% rate in 2014 (Berlin Institute for Population and Development 2014: 48).

According to Kafeero and Birungi (2014), Uganda topped the child dependency ratio (ie number of children per 100 persons of working age) in Eastern Africa at 97, second only to Niger for all of Africa at 106 per 100 working adults (Kafeero and Birungi 2014: 32, Figure 21). The figure for Mozambique was 88 and that for Ethiopia, due in part to its strong contraceptive planning, was 77.[4] Additional factors

---

[4]   The United Nations Population Fund (UNFPA 2011) links the high youth dependency ratio to a lack of gender equality for women, notably, early or child marriage, along with peer pressure from husbands and extended family: "In rural areas of the country, many women become dependent on men, not by choice or longstanding tradition, but by default through the practice of lobolo, where a man offers gifts or money to a woman's parents in exchange for a bride. And once the man pays for the bride, he expects her to have children who can work on the farm or help out with household chores." In addition, for Mozambique and many other states, "early marriage, which is associated with high fertility, is more common among girls with little or no education. The Government outlawed marriage before the age of 16, and since 2004 when a new Family Law went into effect, a child may not marry before reaching 18 without parental consent. But the law is difficult to enforce, particularly in remote areas." Furthermore, among women

identified in the report include access to education for women, thus overcoming pressure for young marriage.

While the number of hospitals with Basic and Comprehensive Emergency Care in Ethiopia is not hugely different from those of the other two countries (at 88), the number of health centers overall with this capability (at 1,813) is impressive (Kafeero and Birungi 2014: 49). The Generation 2030 report also observes that 2,366 professionals had been trained to provide these services. Unfortunately, the national average for skilled attendants helping at birth is still low (at 15%), and the disparity between rural and urban areas actually grew from 2000 to 2014 (Kafeero and Birungi 2014: 51). Ethiopia has made great strides in its social sectors but needs to improve the percentage of skilled attendants helping at deliveries.

Note, in particular, the disparity involving urban and rural locations. This can be explained at least to some degree, of course, as a function of resource availability. However, it is also possible that the greater persistence of traditional beliefs—especially in a state with the topography of Ethiopia—could explain the ability of quite patriarchal views to persist in remote areas virtually unchanged for a very long time. This could work to the disadvantage of women's reproductive health, in particular, because it intersects with inherently controversial subjects such as the use of contraceptives.

Another aspect of the evidence amassed for this book, with hope for influencing its readers, is the enormous importance of multilevel, supranational mechanisms and alliances for bringing changes to traditional African practices when they are harmful to health. One hugely important supranational lever has been the formulation of the MDGs, particularly MDGs 2–6. At the same time of the formulation of the MDGs in 2000, the Global Vaccine Alliance (GAVI) was formed, with 21% of its funding coming from private organizations, the largest being the Gates Foundation.

Without the spur of the world's focus on the MDGs and the funding available through those mechanisms, quite simply, the plight of the marginalized (mainly rural and refugee women and children) would not have changed. While international religious organizations such as World Vision are helpful—since their aid comes without strings

---

in Mozambique without formal education, "only about 1 in 10 women uses a contraceptive, while nearly 4 in 10 women with at least a secondary education uses contraceptives.... The fertility rate in the capital, where women are generally more educated and have easier access to contraception, is three, about half the national average."

attached to client behavior—this is less likely to be true for religious organizations *per se*. The history of these organizations in promoting the status quo in male sexual behavior needed to be countered by secular groups that could take a step back and discuss, for example, the need for increased birth control, sexual health information, and abortion availability to women who rarely had control in these areas. Thus, as we have noted in the country chapters, the most pronounced changes with respect to the MDGs has been in reducing the male–female enrollment disparity, particularly in urban primary schools. Secondary schools have seen some progress along these lines, but in keeping with the relatively recent time period of the MDGs, male–female literacy gaps will take longer to change. Health-care disparities based on gender can therefore be expected to persist.

Decreases in child mortality under MDG 4 have been brought about by the presence of the GAVI providing malarial vaccines and other vaccines to babies and youngsters in Africa. Also, the global project to reduce infant and child mortality due to HIV infection had a large role to play. It is recognized that MDGs 4–6 are intertwined since the circumstances in which a mother lives and gives birth are connected to the life chances of her infant. Thus, research shows that two of the three most prevalent causes for infant death are either lack of prenatal care or intra-partum issues (at birth); the third is pneumonia.

Reduction in malarial infections and other diseases came about due to the leadership efforts of the United Nations Children's Fund (UNICEF) and the GAVI, along with the MDG structure, as well as those of some religious organizations. It goes without saying, however, that the "no condom support" policy practiced by religious organizations is incapable of reducing sexually transmitted diseases and HIV infection.

Based on an international focus through the MDGs and work by pro-choice groups, all three countries, but especially Ethiopia, liberalized their abortion availability over the first decade of the 21st century. A related reduction in maternal mortality has been seen in Ethiopia and in Mozambique, where, in addition to Uganda, unsafe abortion has been a major cause of maternal mortality.

Regional efforts to reduce health gaps between the marginalized and those with power have also been crucial to progress, especially in closing disparities related to women's health. The Maputo Protocol to the African Charter adopted in 2003 and the most recent element of the effort to decriminalize abortion announced by the African Commission on Human and People's Rights in 2016 stand out in that sense. The presence of the Maputo Protocol and the focus it gives to international groups to convey the lack of acceptability of FGM in the

21st century have had some success, but, as discussed in the country chapters, there is a way to go. Ethiopia is a country marked by some of the highest FGM rates in the world and Mozambique has seen an increase due to refugees from FGM-practicing countries. As discussed for Uganda, while FGM is outlawed, certain groups in Eastern Uganda are still practicing it. The practice seems to depend less on religion as much as a connection to traditional ways of life, especially in rural areas. This is a potentially important finding; even among populations with adherents to more Western religious tendencies, FGM still occurs at a high rate.

With regard to another element of women's vulnerability, there has been a large regional and supranational effort in the 21st century to make child marriage (ie under 18) illegal. The rate has dropped in all three countries but not yet enough to make it extinct. Again, the issues with child marriage cycle back to MDGs 4 and 5, especially in terms of extremely young mothers, who often experience horrific physical problems, such as fistula due to long, obstructed labor and infant death during birth.

Some who favor a traditionalist view of relationships between the sexes, notably, those of conservative religious faiths, are skeptical about the impact of supranational mechanisms and funding under the MDGs and other initiatives upon African society. Others understand that too much of the African populace is not able to realize its full potential due to being kidnapped, being forced to bear children at an early age, suffering FGM, having a lack of agency in reproductive health, or having unequal access to education. Those readers in this category will find the emphasis on regional and supranational mechanisms helpful to providing political will and funding to change traditionalist practices. This is also the view taken by those in feminist health politics, such as the volumes authored by Haussman (2005) and Boyd-Judson and James (2013). Those adhering to the view that "women's rights are human rights," first articulated at the Vienna Conference on Human Rights in 1993 and often repeated by many others, understand the central importance of judgment-free sexual and reproductive health care to a woman's full autonomy. In this sense, the tension between traditional values, promoted by some religions or local groups, has been overcome by exposure to secular values and funding.

Summing up

Points of intuition about health in African states, put forward in Chapter 1, are affirmed by the research carried out in this project. These points of intuition refer to processes and outcomes, respectively.

First, religion is significant for the processes of the provision and consumption of health care. Activity from Faith-Based Organizations in provision reflects the excess of the demand over supply of health care from respective governments. With regard to consumption, belief systems make people ready to pursue health in a holistic way—spiritual and physical needs are regarded as connected. Health services provision and consumption in the three states seems quite rational, aside from destructive exceptions involving witchcraft and some other religious beliefs that interfere with optimal health care under resource constraints.

Second, when viewed from the standpoint of women's health in particular, outcomes reveal nuances not obvious upon initial inspection. The MDGs show improvement for Uganda, Mozambique, and Ethiopia. At the same time, gender-related gaps in health outcomes work to the disadvantage of women. These differences reflect, at least in part, the impact of traditional and religious values in each respective society.

With regard to MDGs 2 and 4–6 for Uganda, Mozambique, and Ethiopia, both progress and lack thereof are detected. Overall, all three countries have ratified the Convention on the Elimination of all Forms of Discrimination Against Women and two of the three have ratified the Maputo Protocol to the African Charter, including its strong statements against FGM and for elective abortion. The latter has recently been emphasized by the African Commission on Human and People's Rights (to which the Charter, including the Maputo Protocol, is attached). On January 18, 2016, the Commission launched a continental campaign for the Decriminalization of Abortion in Africa. At the time, it was noted that of the 57 member states, 25 had either blanket prohibitions on the procedure or only allowed it to save the mother's life (International Justice Resource Center 2016). This category does not describe the three countries in this volume. Uganda, Mozambique, and Ethiopia have broadened the conditions under which abortion is decriminalized since the first decade of the MDGs. As previously discussed, this is likely due, at least in part, to international pressure under MDG 5a to reduce by three quarters the maternal mortality ratio by 2015.

With respect to MDG 2 and the goal that by 2015, all boys and girls will be able to complete primary school, the three countries have shown progress. This is also true for MDG 3.1, with an increase for the ratio of girls to boys in primary, secondary, and tertiary education. By 2013, the Uganda country report on the MDGs showed 80% of boys and girls enrolled in primary school. However, the figures became more sex-skewed at the higher levels of education, with young women at 85% of the male figure in secondary school and 79% at the tertiary level. The Uganda MDG report also stated that, among 15–24 year olds in Uganda in 2010, 77% of young men were literate versus 75% for women. In Mozambique, primary school enrollment jumped to 81% by 2010 (Republic of Mozambique 2010). However, the boy–girl ratio in attending and completing different levels of schooling is complicated by wealth, regional, and rural–urban divides. The report stated that female illiteracy had declined to 56% by 2009. On many measures, such as education and maternal health, Ethiopia appears to have taken the MDGs most seriously among the countries in this study. Perhaps that is because it is the second most populous country in Africa and needs international funding intensely. In any event, analysis of Ethiopia in Chapter 5 reveals progress. Note the more than trebled number of previous primary school builds between 1994 and 2014 (Ethiopia 2014). Ethiopia shares with Mozambique a disparity, interacting with gender and wealth differences, between urban and rural access to education. While there are basically 1:1 ratios of attendance between boys and girls at urban primary and secondary schools in Mozambique and Ethiopia, there is only about 5% attendance in rural Ethiopia. Unfortunately, a large literacy gap persists between Ethiopian men and women—up to 20%.

MDGs 4 (reduce child mortality), 5 (improve maternal health), and 6 (combat HIV/AIDS, malaria, and other diseases) are influenced by the nature of conservative policymaking in the three African states, along with the prevalence of religious and customary law in various areas. Inter-group and inter-border tensions are unfortunately still evident in Mozambique and Ethiopia, as are large refugee camps. These are relevant factors because they indicate not only social turmoil, but also, in particular, the abduction of child "brides" (ie married before age 18). While all three countries have laws against marriage before 18, they are not always enforced, especially in rural areas under customary law. Thus, as noted in Chapter 4, Mozambique has the 10th-highest rate of child marriage in the world and the rate in Uganda is quite high as well. Among the ramifications of child marriage are that young women are physically and mentally unprepared to have children. With inconsistent access to prenatal care, especially outside the big cities, young women give birth in the least fortuitous circumstances. While the three countries under study have increased the availability of trained birth attendants, Chapter 5 shows that it can be hard to get women to go to the facilities where they exist. However, interventions such as bringing their traditional food accompaniments and healers can make more of them amenable to going to a modern facility.

Uganda, Mozambique, and Ethiopia still have a long way to go vis-a-vis the MDGs and related objectives: Uganda still has an unacceptably high unsafe abortion rate; Mozambique has unacceptably low contraceptive rates and high child marriage rates; and Ethiopia has unacceptably high rates of FGM, with a staggering majority of women in the country reporting having been subjected to the procedure. On the positive side, it is clear that: (1) maternal mortality ratios due to unsafe abortion (and being under the watch of the MDG partners and money) have been in decline; and (2) child HIV infections have been reduced—these are two of the success stories in the three countries. Adult HIV infections and AIDS are harder to combat, especially if condoms are not used. Formerly, all three countries had staggeringly high maternal mortality ratios: Ethiopia of 1,400 per 100,000 live births in 1990, and Uganda of over 500 and Mozambique of over 600 in the early part of the new millennium. All have reduced their rates—not at the three quarters envisioned by MDG 5a, but showing progress.

Uneasy tension between access to education, jobs, wealth, and health care in urban versus rural areas is pronounced in all three countries. As also demonstrated in Chapters 3–5, people with education are more familiar with, and willing to use, family planning to avert a birth rate that is unacceptable for a family and physically dangerous to the would-be mother. Ethiopia has made huge strides in the treatment of, and education about, obstetric fistula, but obviously more needs to happen. While Ethiopia has national laws against rape and child marriage, it needs to do more to implement them. Ethiopia should also join Mozambique and Uganda in ratifying the Maputo Protocol against FGM. Similarly, girls need not fear going to school due to menstruation or be pulled out of school by being married at a too-early age.

It is clear that the various multi-level instruments, including the MDGs (and now the Sustainable Development Goals), the Global Plan to eliminate new HIV infections among children, the Maputo Protocol, and the Africa Women's Decade 2010–2020, have all helped to empower groups seeking to get national governments either to allow women full reproductive rights access (as envisioned in the 1995 Beijing Platform) or to at least implement their own laws on the books. As with the global faith communities, the pro-reproductive and sexual rights communities have done much to help Africa, including the three states under study here, but there remain a lot of steps yet to take.

This volume has attempted to explain how Africans both provide and secure health care, responding to the physical, mental, and spiritual needs of individuals seeking restoration. Africans have, of course, had health-care policies long before the introduction of modern, Western-style health care beginning with Christian missions in the latter part of the 19th century. In both state and stateless societies in pre-colonial Africa, individuals and institutions existed to supply needed services. Both the colonial era and the independence era introduced vast changes to health-care policies on the continent. New entrants, ideas, and technologies transformed the ways in which Africans supplied and demanded health care. Christian missionary organizations and the state—in both the colonial and independence eras—introduced policies to meet the health-care needs of citizens. These policies, in turn, continue to affect the behavior of Africans.

A conceptual model of religion and health care in Africa

From the outset, this study has taken a decidedly inductive approach. With a focus on just three out of 55 states in Africa, it is prudent to view the research as generating rather than testing explanations for the role of religion regarding health care in Africa. At the same time, it is appropriate to give some attention to the possible contents of a conceptual model. It almost goes without saying that all of what follows will be subject to revision as research accumulates.

Developments reported in this volume have modified, but not completely supplanted, the traditional means and understandings of health care that existed previously. As this book has demonstrated, changes over time have created a complex interaction of many elements that comprise health care. In assessing policy implications for health care in Africa, it is thus important to understand the various elements that comprise both the structure and the processes of this complex whole.

Figure 6.1 illustrates the complex interplay of supply and demand that constitutes health care in Africa. The two main elements endogenous to the model, lying within Africa itself, are the state and civil society. Civil society has been disaggregated for the purposes of health care into providers who are: (1) traditional in their beliefs and approach; and (2) more modern, which can and does include both Christians and Muslims. Africans, of course, both supply and demand health care for themselves. Demand for health care is mediated by financial means, the beliefs of those seeking health care, and their distance from supply. These factors, as seen in the three case chapters, affect health-seeking behaviors.

State and civil society do, of course, interact. The state provides both resources and the policy and legal framework under which all health-care delivery exists. Nonetheless, it is important to note that states in Africa possess relatively less capacity to deliver services compared to more economically developed countries. This limitation has meant, in practical terms, a greater reliance on civil society organizations to deliver needed services. This is true not only in the health-care policy area, but others as well, most notably, education. Despite this weakness, the state retains levers with which to influence health-care policies. As seen in Mozambique and Ethiopia, the state may actively seek to suppress civil society or non-state actors providing health care. The state may also seek to cooperate with, or co-opt, such providers. Current policies in the three countries examined in this volume demonstrated a high degree of cooperation.

This study also shows that faith-based health-care suppliers cooperate with one another. In Ethiopia, for example, Protestant and Muslim health-care providers offer contraception services to Roman Catholics—a fact not unknown to Roman Catholic leadership. Relatively less cooperation took place between traditional and Christian/Muslim faith-based health-care providers, at least in terms

Figure 6.1: A conceptual model of religion and health care in Africa

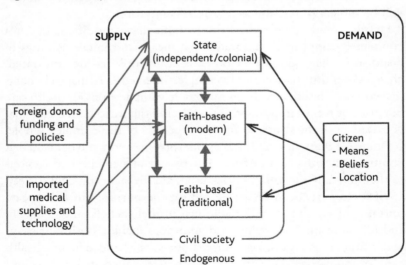

184

of formal mechanisms. Informally, however, all parties interviewed knew about the actions of the other.

Cultural beliefs and actions provide a dynamic to these structural elements. Africans, like people elsewhere in the world, seek health care to obtain or sustain good health. In the case of Africa, beliefs of people mediate how this happens. Africans understand the physical dynamics of health, but also affirm its spiritual realities. In other words, a strictly materialist world view associated with modern, scientific medicine is rejected by Africans. Governments, for the most part, accept this world view and behavior, with the proviso that citizens also obtain access to modern medicine. As seen in Mozambique, the government worked with traditional healers to identify deadly diseases such as malaria and HIV/AIDS that could be referred to modern health clinics. On the other hand, the government ignored the spiritual aspects of traditional healing. An interesting dynamic also emerged for Pentecostal and traditional African beliefs. Both groups agreed on an underlying spiritual cause of poor health, along with the need to address that challenge in seeking services concerned with physical health, but they had disagreements on the legitimacy of spiritual contacts. The state, for its part, saw emphasis on the spiritual as hindering the efficacy of diagnosis and treatment using modern medicine.

Exogenous to the model are actors outside the state and civil society. These are of three types: states actors, intergovernmental organizations, and NGOs. These actors reflect their own interests and aims with respect to the recipient state. African states are relatively undeveloped compared to others, so they have been influenced by parties outside the state. One of the major methods has been through foreign assistance. With aid comes conditionality, which essentially consists of expectations for domestic policies that conform to the wishes of the donor. The HIV/AIDS pandemic, for example, led to state and governmental aid to fund policies for prevention and treatment. The US has contributed billions of dollars for such health-care policies through the US President's Emergency Plan for AIDS Relief (PEPFAR). The comingling of faith-based health-care delivery organizations and foreign aid has itself proven challenging due to political norms within the US regarding the state funding of religious organizations and the concerns of such entities that their religious mission would be abridged by government regulation.

For intergovernmental organizations such as the UN and the European Union, the importance of the MDGs underscores that such organizations have interests and expectations. They, too, interact with faith-based health-care delivery organizations, as seen in Ethiopia,

Mozambique, and Uganda. In such cases, cultural and social norms expected by such organizations may clash with local norms. This is observed on issues such as contraception, abortion, homosexuality, and social relations in general.

A third category of foreign donors consists of NGOs. These organizations are the delivery mechanisms for health care from funders such as states and intergovernmental bodies. They have interests and agendas as well. It is clear from the research that these organizations have played an important role in the supply of health care. Some are themselves faith-based. Here, too, religious belief, in this case, on the part of the leaders and missions of such organizations, affect the delivery of health care. For example, in Ethiopia, Lutheran leaders expressed concern over the ending of funding of their hospitals due to donor disagreement with their views on same-sex marriage.

The role of donors and religion in health-care delivery points out that what African states address through policies that reflect the views of their citizens is also affected by the international context in which they exist and their relative weakness. Many of these policies are more secular and materialist in philosophical orientations, which underscores the importance of such donors themselves being sensitive to the religious beliefs of Africans and how this, in turn, affects the provision and demand for health care.

What, then, are the policy implications of this conceptual model? First, it is necessary but not sufficient to focus solely on health care. This approach not only overlooks the cultural and religious beliefs and actions of Africans, but also assumes that the state and foreign donors are themselves neutral. As seen in Chapters 3–5, such actors themselves carry assumptions and attitudes. Thus, it is important not to dismiss religious belief as somehow a hindrance to achieving the MDGs, but to accept that they should guide health-care delivery in such a way that is both effective and respectful of African religious beliefs. The three case studies show that African governments, after having embraced earlier policies that sought to marginalize such faith-based approaches, have changed these policies to work with organizations to achieve common health-care goals.

Second, faith-based and modern health-care delivery systems are complex and dynamic. It is important to understand the distinctions between traditional African, Muslim, and mainline Christian health care—including the differences between Protestant Evangelical, Roman Catholic, and Pentecostal understandings and approaches. "Faith-based/faith-inspired" is a useful broad category in which to lump civil society organizations that share a religious motivation for their work in health care, but policies must then move to greater specificity and understanding to be more effective in delivery. Again, as revealed by the three case studies, African governments are cognizant of these differences and generally work with Faith-Based Organizations to achieve their goals. One possible exception is noted in Mozambique, where the government and a major and influential Pentecostal denomination lack mechanisms to connect with one another on common goals. Theologically, Pentecostalism is Anabaptist, which generally posits a strong divergence between the church and state, lessening the connection between the two. For its part, the government of Mozambique appeared frustrated with the denomination's health-care views. This case is important because Pentecostalism is a growing movement on the continent. As Pentecostalism grows in influence, it will be increasingly important to foster ties between these church bodies and the broader public via the state.

Despite any number of challenges, substantial progress has been made over the past two decades in addressing the health-care needs of the continent. On many metrics, the quality of health for Africans has improved, despite a very rapid growth in population. This latter point is not fully appreciated. As Africa grows in population and wealth, the policies, understandings, and approaches of Africans will increasingly come to bear on international debates regarding the provision of health care. This will include the experiences of Africans in reconciling the various elements examined in this book inherent in the supply of and demand for health care in Africa, most notably, religious belief. A time can thus be foreseen when a sensitivity to religious belief and health care is part of the agenda for other states and international organizations such as the UN.

Along those lines, need remains for the various actors in the provision of health care to interact more frequently and deeply. The conceptual analysis of this book in terms of African Studies, Religious Studies, and Health Studies (ie the overlapping fields depicted in Figure 2.1) pointed out that these three areas are separate silos in theory and in practice. The boundaries of these three conceptual domains for those who are sick and those who provide health care, however, are not so neatly drawn. Africans operate within a complex interaction of beliefs, ideology, science, experience, governments, civil society organizations, health care, and trust. Africans themselves are not always certain of the boundaries between belief and science.

Within Chapter 5 on Ethiopia, an interviewee from the HIV/AIDS Prevention and Control Office spoke positively of cooperative efforts between government and religious organizations against HIV/AIDS.

Importantly, this official noted that among such religious organizations, "territories" existed. An example is the use of condoms. Thus, even with Faith-Based Organizations, there are boundaries. This echoed the integrative approach observed by Slikkerveer (1982: 1860–1861).

For Mozambique in Chapter 4, the boundaries of the domains are different. The Director of Traditional Medicine in that country envisioned a public health model where physical needs would be met by modern medicine and emotional, mental, and spiritual needs by religious believers. This was not, however, the way traditional healers and leaders in the emerging churches understood the boundaries. In comparison, for Uganda in Chapter 3, boundaries are observed on the provision side of the equation as relatively less coordinated and integrative, particularly for traditional medicine.

While there is awareness, cooperation, and respect, the policy challenge is the existence of misunderstanding and even mistrust. A major policy implication is to continue efforts to foster the types of cooperative efforts observed in all three countries. This is probably most critical for the interaction between governments/international organizations and Africa's traditional healers/emerging churches. It is between these groups and modern medicine that the biggest gap in understanding and cooperation continues.

This need for deliberative efforts to seek areas of mutual understanding and agreement extends to scholar, practitioners, and international organizations as well. This is not to say that no efforts have previously been undertaken, but to point out that research shows significant gaps in interaction among all of the actors in the provision of health care. Indeed, such deliberate interactions to address differences of analytical approach and the assessment of research became necessary even among the authors of this book, who themselves reflect a variety of academic and health backgrounds. The complexity of health care and religion in Africa requires this paradoxical willingness to both affirm and set aside approaches and identifications to understand its processes, structures, and outcomes. Some final thoughts on this are presented in Chapter 7.

7

Conclusion

Overview

With a focus on three states in Eastern Africa, this study has examined the role of religion in health-care processes and outcomes. The results can be summarized as religion matters.

Results affirm the frame of reference offered by the Social Determinants of Health with regard to processes. Religion is significant for processes concerning the provision and consumption of health care. Faith-based entities are important, even essential, in health care for Uganda, Mozambique, and Ethiopia. Moreover, health-seeking behavior is impacted upon by a holistic mindset in which physical and mental health are intertwined. Africans thus pursue health care in a rational way, given their world view, with openness to and even preference for faith-based provision under circumstances in which government efforts fall short of basic needs. A review of health outcomes, centered around the Millennium Development Goals, reveals progress across the board. Attention to women's health, however, reveals nuances in the generally upward-shifting values for the Millennium Development Goals. Religious and traditional belief systems play at least some role in holding back outcomes for women relative to men, and exacerbating problems frequently connected with the inherently contested area of reproductive health.

These findings are in line with the rigorous but relatively limited academic literature, reviewed in Chapter 2, on health care in Africa. Health-seeking behavior in the three states included here confirms a holistic way of thinking that blends the physical and spiritual together. Faith-based providers, in line with such preferences and the inadequate performance by governments, represent a significant component of health. Interviews and other data on Uganda, Mozambique, and Ethiopia do nothing to change the sense that any comparative advantage for faith-based providers of health care remains open to question. These entities tend to offer the same services as government-run facilities. Quite certain after a review of the evidence is the focus by faith-based health-care providers on HIV/AIDS and service to the poor. In sum, the previous foundation of research on the role of religion in health for Africa is confirmed by the case studies of Uganda, Mozambique, and Ethiopia carried out here.

This chapter unfolds in two further sections. The first section focuses on implications for concept formation and interdisciplinary fields. The second offers ideas about causal inference, methods, and other research priorities.

Implications for concept formation and interdisciplinary academic fields

Consider first the concepts of Africa, religion, and health, which were introduced in Chapter 1. Evidence from just three states is enough to confirm the diversity of Africa in terms of its people, terrain, and other characteristics.

Upon the conclusion of the research, it still seems appropriate to continue the practice of staying away from a formal definition of religion. Some belief systems commonly identified as religions, such as Islam and Christianity, are found in each of the three states under review. Traditional belief systems—commonly but perhaps misleadingly labeled as "animism"—also persist, though at lower levels than in the past. Witchcraft, fortunately now quite limited in appeal, probably falls outside the boundaries of religion and more within the boundaries of cult-like behavior.

Research in this volume affirms the concept formation at the outset regarding Africa. The continent is at once undergoing change along numerous dimensions that, collectively speaking, amount to dramatic modernization. Health care is no exception. At the same time, the importance of traditional belief systems, notably, those linked to religion, persists. Africans are at once modern and traditional, with the health field perhaps identifying the continent as the one from around the world that most strongly stands out in such a hybrid way.

Results obtained from interviews complement prior research in supporting the Social Determinants of Health as an informative way in which to understand the concept of health. The holistic sense of health among Africans is reaffirmed on many occasions in prior chapters. Health is understood by Africans in a comprehensive way that includes religion in terms of both supply and demand. All of this is very much in line with the perspective adopted from the Social Determinants of Health.

What about the interdisciplinary fields of Religious Studies, African Studies, and Health Studies? Implications for these fields, which were introduced in Chapter 1 to help set the context for the study, are considered in turn.

With respect to Religious Studies, the present study leans toward a positivist approach, but not without attention to phenomenological or self-generated understanding. Interviewees spoke of their faith, at times, in a transcendent way. The interviewers probed beneath the surface meaning of the words used in order to learn as much as possible about the health process along the way. Sensitivity to context, given the research team's prior experience in Africa, facilitated such understanding. Perhaps the current project can be summed up as one that tries to "thread the needle" between the positivist's call for objective evidence and the phenomenologist's prioritizing of dialogue and mutual understanding within a context. This study includes both quantitative data on Millennium Development Goals and interview-based material, so at least in principle it represents a balanced approach to the religiously oriented subject matter.

From the standpoint of African Studies, the present study is also balanced in approach. It is area-oriented—consistent with the African Studies tradition—and also quite interdisciplinary. For example, a link with gender studies is maintained throughout the review of the Millennium Development Goals as measurements of outcomes. More nuanced interpretations result from the standpoint of women's health in reviewing improvements at the national level—women, in short, sometimes end up lagging behind in health outcomes. Another interdisciplinary link is with economics, albeit in a non-technical way. No equations are used, but the concepts of supply and demand are borrowed to facilitate analysis and provide at least part of the explanation for why Faith-Based Organizations are so prominent in the provision of health care. Africans emerge as rational actors within this frame of reference.

With regard to Health Studies, the Social Determinants of Health framework is strongly affirmed by the present investigation of religion and health in three African states. As noted many times already, religion is essential to both the provision and consumption of health care. The social element in health care receives support from the evidence available through the assessment of religion's role in Uganda, Mozambique, and Ethiopia.

Causal inference, methods, and other research priorities

Given the nature of this study, with just three states, it is obvious that inferences about the role of religion regarding health care in Africa as a whole are not justified. Instead, the exercise is intended as one to generate ideas and even hypotheses for testing as more data become available. Figure 6.1, which conveyed a conceptual model of religion and health care in Africa, is a step in that direction. Given the diversity of Africa, there is some justification in continuing an inductive approach in some additional cases, at least to the point at which a representative sample of the continent's 57 states is reached.[1] It clear that the role of religion is mixed, with some positive and negative elements identified and variation among the three states included so far. Some of the most positive elements pertain to the provision of services by Faith-Inspired Institutions. The most negative aspects tend to come through when assessing outcomes, conveyed through Millennium Development Goals, when special attention is paid to women's health.

One of the most positive aspects of the current study is its ability to generate a wide range of ideas for subsequent research projects. Possible new directions, in no presumed order of importance, are enumerated at this point.

Perhaps the most obvious pathway concerns expansion of the sample to other African states. Most notable is the absence of any Muslim-majority states, among approximately 20 in Africa, in the existing sample of Uganda, Mozambique, and Ethiopia. Islam and Christianity differ along multiple dimensions: structure, level of strictness, engagement in civil society, histories in relation to colonization, and views of women and reproductive health. All of that could impact upon the role of religion within the provision and consumption of health care for a given state. Consider, for example, Nigeria, the largest state in Africa, within which Muslims are a majority. Does Nigeria fit the pattern of this book? Are Muslims in Nigeria more likely to be suspicious of Western medicine? What about the role of outside actors in this context? More specifically, are states from the Middle East more active than the West in health care for Nigeria and other Muslim-majority countries? It would be especially interesting to study the Gulf States in this context. All of the preceding questions are both interesting and important to answer.

Another obvious gap in the research concerns religion, religious practices, and religious competition. Interesting questions arise in this context: why would more religious people (or those who belong

[1] It is important to bear in mind that some specialists in African Studies would prefer not to include the north of Africa, that is, less than 57 states would be deemed relevant for purposes of generalization. This matter is beyond the scope of the current exposition, which focuses directly on three states from sub-Saharan Africa.

to stricter religions, like Pentecostalism) be more disposed to comply with health-related restrictions? What are the potential roles of social control, socialization, and social learning? These queries, collectively speaking, should also be a priority to answer.

Methodological triangulation, if resources become available, would also enhance understanding and explanation of the role of religion in health for Africa. The present investigation has relied upon interviews and publicly available compilations of statistics, such as those for the Millennium Development Goals. In the future, techniques such as surveys, survey experiments, and statistical analyses would be desirable to implement. If quantitative and qualitative results then exhibit consistency with each other, confidence in the tentative conclusions offered here would naturally increase. Research could also encompass states beyond Africa to see if at least some of the patterns identified for the role of religion in health care hold up even beyond its boundaries.

Even more broadly, disciplines beyond those incorporated in the present study can be accessed for insights. Consider, for instance, economics, which already has a valuable academic literature that applies principles from rational choice to explain the role of religion in the contemporary world (Iannacone 1994, 1995; Iannacone et al 1998). A rational choice perspective can help to account for how and why competition contributes to religious growth. Such studies also account for variation in the strength of religion on a geographic basis, with Africa and the Middle East versus Western Europe as the most graphic comparison. From a rational choice standpoint, people seek to maximize benefits and minimize costs. Benefits from religious affiliation include a sense of belonging to family and beyond, services of various kinds, and a feeling of security derived from belief in an afterlife (Iannaccone 1994, 1995; Iannaccone et al 1998).

Finally, religion might be investigated in connection with a wider range of issues. It is already certain that religion impacts upon health. However, does religion also matter with respect to education, security, and other issues? This study encourages such investigations. In addition, these issues might be investigated in a wider network—perhaps security, religion, and health might be a starting point—to identify more complex interactions between and among them. In that sense, health could be investigated in the roles of both cause and effect in the quest for more comprehensive knowledge about this essential element of life.

Appendix

Interviewees, affiliations, and dates for Uganda

Interview	Date
Doctor who works with Ministry of Health	March 2, 2012
Politician	February 29, 2012
Worker at health centre	March 1, 2012
Program specialist	March 2, 2012
Employee, Ministry of Health	March 2, 2012
Professor	March 4, 2012
Politician	January 22, 2013
Doctor (and colleagues) at Ministry of Health	January 22, 2013
Government official	March 1, 2012
Government official	February 29, 2012
District health officer	March 1, 2012
Health consultant	September 4, 2013
Professor	February 29, 2012
HIV program, faith-based lead	March 2, 2012
Herbalist/witch doctor	January 23, 2013
Employee, Health Centre III	January 23, 2013
Village traditional birth attendant (in their home, through a translator)	January 23, 2013
Professor and doctor	February 29, 2012
Hospital administrator	March 2, 2012
Employee, Health Center IV	January 23, 2013
Employee, health centre	January 23, 2013
Employee, health centre (Catholic hospital)	January 23, 2013

Interviews and dates for Mozambique

Interviews	Date
Officer, USAID in Mozambique	June 28, 2011
Officer, Ministry of Health	June 23, 2011
Administrator, Ministry of Health	June 27, 2011
Official, Igreja Universal do Reino de Deus	June 28, 2011
Official, Presbyterian Church of Mozambique	June 23, 2011
Employee, World Vision, Mozambique	June 27, 2011
Member, Comunidade Muçulmano: Acção Humanitária	June 28, 2011
Employee, World Vision, Mozambique	June 27, 2011
Employee, Inhaca Clinic	June 25, 2011
Pastor, Maputo International Christian Fellowship	June 26, 2011
Officials, Traditional Medicine, Ministry of Health	June 24, 2011

Interviewees, affiliations and dates for Ethiopia

Interview	Date
Professor, Addis Ababa University	May 15, 2014
Official, HIV/AIDS Prevention and Control Office	May 15, 2014
Professor, Addis Ababa University	May 13, 2014
Official, The Ethiopian Evangelical Church, Mekane Yesus	May 13, 2014
Official, Consortium on Christian Relief and Development Association (CCRDA), NCA	May 16, 2014
MD, The Ethiopian Evangelical Church, Mekane Yesus	May 13, 2014
Official, CCRDA	May 16, 2014
Member, Ethiopian Orthodox Church	May 15, 2014
Official, CCRDA, Christian Aid	May 16, 2014
Official, CCRDA	May 16, 2014
Official, CCRDA	May 16, 2014
MD, EKC Church	May 13, 2014
Official, CCRDA	May 16, 2014
Official, CCRDA	May 16, 2014
PhD candidate, School of Social Work, Addis Ababa University	May 13, 2014
Official, Ministry of Health	May 14, 2014
Professor, Addis Ababa University	May 16, 2014
Professor, School of Social Work, Addis Ababa University	May 13, 2014
Official, CCRDA	May 16, 2014
Official, CCRDA, program coordinator	May 16, 2014
Professor, School of Public Health, Addis Ababa University	May 14, 2014
Official, The Ethiopian Evangelical Church, Mekane Yesus	May 13, 2014
Official, Development and Inter-Church Aid Commission (three others present)	May 16, 2014
Official, CCRDA, Rev	May 16, 2014
Official, Health and Nutrition, World Vision Ethiopia	May 12, 2014
Official, The Ethiopian Evangelical Church, Mekane Yesus	May 13, 2014
Official, Ethiopian Catholic Secretariat	May 15, 2014
Professor, School of Public Health, Addis Ababa University	May 14, 2014
Member, EKC Church	May 13, 2014
Official, Ethiopian Catholic Secretariat	May 15, 2014
Official, CCRDA	May 16, 2014
Official, HIV/AIDS Prevention and Control Office	May 15, 2014
Team members, rural health center	May 16, 2014

Demographic summary for Ethiopia and Uganda

Uganda and Ethiopia are both multi-ethnic societies, with recent histories marked by civil war and military dictatorship. Since the 1960s both countries have experienced rapid population growth. Uganda accounted for around 7.2 million individuals at independence in 1962. However, 50 years later, the total population had risen almost 4.5 times to nearly 33.5 million. In much the same way, Ethiopia's population was estimated at roughly 22.5 million at the start of the 1960s but had risen by almost 3.5 times to almost 83 million in 2010.... Whilst the Ethiopian population has grown more in absolute numbers, Uganda's comparatively smaller population has been increasing at a much faster rate. Indeed, the growth rate has remained at more than 3 percent since the mid-1970s and Uganda currently has one of the highest growth rates in Sub-Saharan Africa. The corresponding situation in Ethiopia is quite different: following a military coup in the mid-1970s, population growth fell by more than a percentage point. The growth rate then recovered and reached a peak of 3.3 percent in the mid-1990s before entering a period of sustained decline.... During the past 15 years, the gap between the two countries' growth rates has increased. In 2010, the Ethiopian population grew 1 percent less than the Ugandan population. To understand these differences, it is particularly important to look at fertility trends. From 1960 until the beginning of the 1990s, fertility rates remained roughly constant in both countries, with women giving birth to an average of seven children during the course of their lives. From the 1990s onwards, Ethiopian fertility fell. By 2010, average fertility in the country was around 2.5 children per woman. In contrast to this, Ugandan fertility only experienced small declines in the same period. In 2010, average fertility remained high at about 6.4 children per woman.

Source: Berlin Institute for Population and Development (2014: 1).

References

28tooMany. 2013. "Country Profile: FGM in Uganda, 2013." Available at: www.28tooMany.org (accessed July 2017).

Abebe, Yigeremu, Ab Schaap, Girmatchew Mamo, Asheber Negussie, Birke Darimo, Dawit Wolday, and Eduard J. Sanders. 2003. "HIV Prevalence in 72,000 Urban and Rural Male Army Recruits, Ethiopia." *AIDS* 17: 1835–1840.

Africa Review. 2017. "Sweden Gives Mozambique $5.2 m for safe abortion," March 2.

African Studies Association. 2016. "About the ASA." Available at: www.africanstudies.org/about-the-asa

African Union. 2010. "List of Countries which Have Signed, Ratified/ Acceded to the Protocol to the African Charter on Human and People's Rights on the Rights of Women in Africa," July 22.

Agadjanian, Victor. 2005. "Gender, Religious Involvement, and HIV/AIDS Prevention in Mozambique." *Social Science & Medicine* 61: 1529–1539. Available at: www.ncbi.nlm.nih.gov/pmc/articles/PMC1781404/

Agadjanian, Victor. 2012. "Religious Organizations and the Fight Against HIV/AIDS in Mozambique." In Jill Olivier and Quentin Wodon (eds) *The Role of Faith-Inspired Health Care Providers in Sub-Saharan Africa and Public–Private Partnerships: Strengthening the Evidence for Faith-Inspired Health Engagement in Africa, Volume 1.* Washington, DC: The World Bank, pp 131–139.

Agadjanian, Victor and Soma Sen. 2007. "Promises and Challenges of Faith-Based AIDS Care and Support in Mozambique." American Journal of Public Health 97(2): 362–366.

Alles, Gregory D. 2008. "Afterword: Toward a Global Vision of Religious Studies." In Gregory D. Alles (ed) *Religious Studies: A Global View.* New York, NY: Routledge, pp 301–322.

Alles, Gregory D. 2010. "The Study of Religions: The Last 50 Years." In John R. Hinnells (ed) *The Routledge Companion to the Study of Religion* (2nd edn). New York, NY: Routledge, pp 39–55.

Almond, Gabriel and Sidney Verba. 1965. *The Civic Culture: Political Attitudes and Democracy in Five Nations, an Analytical Study.* Boston, MA: Little, Brown.

Almond, Gabriel, Scott Appleby, and Emmanuel Sivan. 2003. *Strong Religion: The Rise of Fundamentalisms Around the World.* Chicago, IL: University of Chicago Press.

Anders, Therese. 2016. *The Influence of Insecurity on Government Welfare Mindedness: Subnational-Level Explorations in Colombia, Indonesia, and Mexico.* Los Angeles, CA: University of Southern California.

Asante, Molefi Kete and Ama Mazama. 2009. *Encyclopedia of African Religion.* Thousand Oaks, CA: SAGE Publications.

ASMEA (Association for the Study of the Middle East and Africa). 2016. "About ASMEA." Available at: www.asmeascholars.org/about/welcome-to-asmea/

Badiani, Rita. 2016. "Advancing Abortion Rights: Lessons from Mozambique," May 11, Pathfinder International. Available at: www.pathfinder.org

Baylies, Carolyn and Janet Bujra (eds). 2000. *AIDS, Sexuality and Gender in Africa: Collective Strategies and Struggles in Tanzania and Zambia.* New York, NY: Routledge.

Becker, M. 1974. *The Health Belief Model and Personal Health Behavior.* Thorofare, NJ: Slack.

Beisheim, Marianne, Andrea Liese, Hannah Janetschek, and Johanna Sarre. 2014. "Transnational Partnerships: Conditions for Successful Service Provision in Areas of Limited Statehood." *Governance: An International Journal of Policy, Administration, and Institutions* 27(4): 655–673.

Berer, Marge. 2017. "Abortion Law and Policy Around the World: In Search of Decriminalization." *Health and Human Rights Journal* 19(1): 13–27.

Berhanu, Zena. 2010. "Holy Water as an Intervention for HIV/AIDS in Ethiopia." *Journal of HIV/AIDS & Social Services* 9: 240–260.

Berlin Institute for Population and Development. 2014. "Realising the Demographic Dividend for Ethiopia and Uganda: A Comparative Analysis." Berlin, Germany.

Birhan, Wubet, Mirutse Giday, and Tilahun Teklehaymanot. 2011. "The Contribution of Traditional Healers' Clinics to Public Health Care System in Addis Ababa, Ethiopia: A Cross-Sectional Study." *Journal of Ethnobiology and Ethnomedicine* 7: 39.

Birhanu, Zewdie, Tsion Assefa, Mirkuzie Woldie, and Sudhakar Morankar. 2012. "Predictors of Perceived Empathy Among Patients Visiting Primary Health-Care Centers in Central Ethiopia." *International Journal for Quality in Health Care* 24(2): 161–168.

Blevins, John, Sandra Thurman, Mimi Kiser, and Laura Beres. 2012. "Community Health Assets Mapping: A Mixed Method Approach in Nairobi." In Jill Olivier and Quentin Wodon (eds) *Mapping, Cost, and Reach to the Poor of Faith-Inspired Health Care Providers in Sub-Saharan Africa: Strengthening the Evidence for Faith-Inspired Health Engagement in Africa, Volume 3*. Washington, DC: The World Bank, pp 91–101.

Boulenger, Delphine, Francoise Barten, and Bart Criel. 2012. "Contracting Between Faith-Based Health Care Organizations and the Public Sector in Sub-Saharan Africa." In Jill Olivier and Quentin Wodon (eds) *The Role of Faith-Inspired Health Care Providers in Sub-Saharan Africa and Public–Private Partnerships: Strengthening the Evidence for Faith-Inspired Health Engagement in Africa, Volume 1*. Washington, DC: The World Bank, pp 60–70.

Boychuck, Gerald. 2008. *National Health Insurance in Canada and the US: Race, Territory and the Roots of Difference*. Washington, DC: Georgetown University Press.

Boyd-Judson, Lyn and Patrick James (eds). 2013. *Women's Global Health: Norms and State Policies*. Lanham, MD: Rowman and Littlefield.

Brown, Adrienne, Mick Foster, Andy Norton, and Felix Naschold. 2001. "Working Paper 142: The Status of Sector Wide Approaches." Centre for Aid and Public Expenditure, January, Overseas Development Institute, London. Available at: www.odi.org/sites/odi.org.uk/files/odi-assets/publications-opinion-files/2071.pdf

Brown, Davis and Patrick James. 2015. "Religious Characteristics of States Dataset." Available at: http://thearda.com/newsearch.asp?searchterms=religious+characteristics+of+states+dataset&c=ABCDEFGHIJKLMNYZ

Budge-Reid, Heather, Donna Asiimve Kusemererwa, and Anke Meiburg. 2012. "Pharmaceutical Service Delivery in Church Health Systems in Africa: A Cross-Country Analysis." In Jill Olivier and Quentin Wodon (eds) *The Role of Faith-Inspired Health Care Providers in Sub-Saharan Africa and Public–Private Partnerships: Strengthening the Evidence for Faith-Inspired Health Engagement in Africa, Volume 1*. Washington, DC: The World Bank, pp 104–117.

Byrne, Peter. 1988. "Religion and the Religions." In Stewart Sutherland and Peter Clarke (eds) *The World's Religions: The Study of Religion, Traditional and New Religion*. London: Routledge, pp 3–28.

Callaghan-Koru, Jennifer A., Abiy Seifu, Maya Tholandi, Joseph de Graft-Johnson, Ephrem Daniel, Barbara Rawlins, Bogale Worku, and Abdullah H. Baqui. 2013. "Newborn Care Practices at Home and in Health Facilities in Four Regions of Ethiopia." *BMC Pediatrics* 13: 198.

Capps, Walter H. 1995. *Religious Studies: The Making of a Discipline*. Minneapolis, MN: Fortress Press.

Capps, Walter H. 2013. "Impressions from Wingspread: Religious Studies—The State of the Art." In Scott S. Elliott (ed) *Reinventing Religious Studies: Key Writings in the History of a Discipline*. Bristol, CT: Acumen, pp 43–45.

Catholic Bishops' Conference of Ethiopia. 2013. *The Ethiopian Catholic Church's Stand on Female Genital Mutilation*. Addis Ababa: Ethiopian Catholic Church.

Cau, Boaventura, Arusyak Sevoyan, and Victor Agadjanian. no date. *Religion, Child Mortality and Health in Mozambique*. Tempe, AZ: Center for Population Dynamics, Arizona State University.

Cau, Boaventura, Arusyak Sevoyan, and Victor Agadjanian. 2013. "Religious Affiliation and under-Five Mortality in Mozambique." *Journal of Biosocial Science* 45(3): 415–429.

Central Statistical Agency (Ethiopia) and ICF International. 2012. *Ethiopia Demographic and Health Survey 2011*. Addis Ababa, Ethiopia, and Calverton, MA: Central Statistical Agency and ICF International. Available at: www.unicef.org/ethiopia/ET_2011_EDHS.pdf

Central Statistical Agency (Ethiopia) and ORC Macro. 2006. *Ethiopia Demographic and Health Survey 2005*. Addis Ababa, Ethiopia and Calverton, MD: Central Statistical Agency and ORC Macro.

Center for Reproductive Rights. 2011. "10 Key Points About Uganda's Laws and Policies on Termination of Pregnancy." Available at: https://www.reproductiverights.org/sites/crr.civicactions.net/files/documents/WEB_pub_fac_uganda_11.28.11.pdf

Centre for Health Sciences Training, Research and Development. 2013. *Fact Sheet on Health and Human Security Approach*. Ibadan, Nigeria: CHESTRAD International.

Chand, Sarla and Jacqui Patterson. 2007. *Faith Based Models for Improving Newborn and Maternal Health*. Maternal and Child Health Division, Office of Health, Infectious Diseases and Nutrition, Bureau for Global Health, and the US Agency for International Development. Available at: http://pdf.usaid.gov/pdf_docs/PNADK571.pdf

Chatlani, Hema. 2006/2007. "Uganda: A Nation in Crisis." *California Western International Law Journal* 37: 277–298.

Chitando, Ezra. 2005. "Phenomenology of Religion and the Study of African Traditional Religions." *Method & Theory in the Study of Religion* 17(4): 299–316.

CIA (Central Intelligence Agency) World Factbook. 2016. Available at: www.cia.gov/library/publications/the-world-factbook/geos/mz.html

Clemens, Michael and Todd Moss. 2005. *What's Wrong with the Millennium Development Goals?* CGD Brief, Washington, DC: Center for Global Development. Available at: www.cgdev.org

Cochrane, James R. 2006. "Conceptualising Religious Health Assets Redemptively." *Religion and Theology* 13(1): 107–120.

Cochrane, James R., Liz Thomas, and Barbara Schmid. 2012. "Masangane: An Integrated Community Response to HIV and AIDS in Rural South Africa." In Jill Olivier and Quentin Wodon (eds) *The Role of Faith-Inspired Health Care Providers in Sub-Saharan Africa and Public–Private Partnerships: Strengthening the Evidence for Faith-Inspired Health Engagement in Africa, Volume 1.* Washington, DC: The World Bank, pp 122–130.

Cooke, Jennifer G. 2009. *Public Health in Africa: A Report of the CSIS Global Health Policy Center.* Washington, DC: Center for Strategic & International Studies.

Coulombe, Harold and Quentin Wodon. 2012a. "Mapping Religious Health Assets: Are Faith–Inspired Facilities Located in Poor Areas in Ghana?" In Jill Olivier and Quentin Wodon (eds) *Mapping, Cost, and Reach to the Poor of Faith-Inspired Health Care Providers in Sub-Saharan Africa: Strengthening the Evidence for Faith-Inspired Health Engagement in Africa, Volume 3.* Washington, DC: The World Bank, pp 62–75.

Coulombe, Harold and Quentin Wodon. 2012b. "Benefit Incidence of Public Health Spending: Comparing Public and Faith-Inspired Providers." In Jill Olivier and Quentin Wodon (eds) *Mapping, Cost, and Reach to the Poor of Faith-Inspired Health Care Providers in Sub-Saharan Africa: Strengthening the Evidence for Faith-Inspired Health Engagement in Africa, Volume 3.* Washington, DC: The World Bank, pp 121–131.

Damtew, Zufan Abera, Chala Tesfaye Chekagn, and Amsalu Shiferaw Moges. 2016. "The Health Extension Program of Ethiopia: Strengthening the Community Health System." *Harvard Health Policy Review*, December 30.

Deneulin, Séverine and Augusto Zampini-Davies. 2017. "Engaging Development and Religion: Methodological Groundings." *World Development* 99: 110–121.

Dieleman, M.A., T. Hilhorst, and J. Utrera. 2012. "Emerging Practices of Faith-Based Organizations Addressing Human Resources for Health." In Jill Olivier and Quentin Wodon (eds) *The Role of Faith-Inspired Health Care Providers in Sub-Saharan Africa and Public–Private Partnerships: Strengthening the Evidence for Faith-Inspired Health Engagement in Africa, Volume 1.* Washington, DC: The World Bank, pp 101–113.

Digby, Anne, Waltraud Ernst, and Prohjit Mukharji (eds). 2010. *Crossing Colonial Historiographies: Histories of Colonial and Indigenous Medicines in Transnational Perspective*. Newcastle: Cambridge Scholars' Press.

Dimmock, Frank, Jill Olivier, and Quentin Wodon. 2012. "Half a Century Young: The Christian Health Associations in Africa." In Jill Olivier and Quentin Wodon (eds) *The Role of Faith-Inspired Health Care Providers in Sub-Saharan Africa and Public–Private Partnerships: Strengthening the Evidence for Faith-Inspired Health Engagement in Africa, Volume 1*. Washington, DC: The World Bank, pp 71–103.

Dube, Francis. 2009. "Colonialism, Cross-Border Movements, and Epidemiology: A History of Public Health in the Manica Region of Central Mozambique and Eastern Zimbabwe and the African Response, 1890–1980," PhD dissertation, University of Iowa. Available at: http://ir.uiowa.edu/etd/2694/

Durr, Benjamin. 2015. "Mozambique Loosens Anti-Abortion Laws." *Aljajzeerh*, January 26. Available at: www.aljazeera.com/indepth/features/2015/01/mozambique-loosens-anti-abortion-laws-150120081246992.html

Egerö, Bertil. 1987. "Mozambique, a Dream Undone: The Political Economy of Democracy, 1975–84." Nordiska afrikainstitutet.

Ethiopia. 2014. *Progress Toward Meeting the Millennium Development Goals*. Addis Ababa: Ministry of Finance and Economic Development.

Ethiopia. October 2015. *Millennium Development Goals Report 2014-Assessment of Ethiopia's Progress Towards the MDG's*. Government of Ethiopia, UN Development Programme, UN Country Team in Ethiopia. Accessed at https://reliefweb.int/report November 5 2018.

Ethiopian Catholic Secretariat Health and HIV/AIDS Unit. 2009. *The Ethiopian Catholic Church Health Policy*. Addis Ababa: Ethiopian Catholic Church.

Ethiopian Civil Society Health Forum. 2013. *Health Forum Newsletter* Edition 1, December.

Ethnologue. 2016a. "Ethnologue: Languages of the World, Uganda." Available at: www.ethnologue.com/country/UG

Ethnologue. 2016b. "Ethnologue: Languages of the World, Ethiopia." Available at: www.ethnologue.com/country/et

FIDH. 2013. "Women's Rights in Africa: 18 Countries Are Yet to Ratify the Maputo Protocol!" Worldwide Movement for Women's Rights. Available at: www.fidh.org (accessed June 24, 2017).

Fistula Foundation. 2017. "Why Do We Work in Ethiopia?" Available at: www.fistulafoundation.org (accessed July 2017).

Foster, Geoff, Talent Maphosa, and Frank Kurebva. 2012. "Faith Untapped: Linking Community-Level and Sectoral Health and HIV/AIDS Responses." In Jill Olivier and Quentin Wodon (eds) *The Comparative Nature of Faith-Inspired Health Care Provision in Sub-Saharan Africa: Strengthening the Evidence for Faith-Inspired Health Engagement in Africa, Volume 2.* Washington, DC: The World Bank, pp 114–120.

Fox, Jonathan. 2008. *A World Survey of Religion and the State.* Cambridge: Cambridge University Press.

Fox, Jonathan. 2013. *An Introduction to Religion and Politics: Theory and Practice.* New York, NY: Routledge.

Fox, Jonathan and Shmuel Sandler. 2004. *Bringing Religion into International Relations.* New York, NY: Palgrave Macmillan.

Freedom House. 2016. *Freedom in the World 2016: Ethiopia.* Available at: https://freedomhouse.org/report/freedom-world/2016/ethiopia

Gemignani, Regina and Quentin Wodon. 2012. "How Do Households Choose Between Health Providers? Results from Qualitative Fieldwork in Burkina Faso." In Jill Olivier and Quentin Wodon (eds) *The Role of Faith-Inspired Health Care Providers in Sub-Saharan Africa and Public–Private Partnerships: Strengthening the Evidence for Faith-Inspired Health Engagement in Africa, Volume 1.* Washington, DC: The World Bank, pp 49–72.

Gemignani, Regina, Clarence Tsimpo, and Quentin Wodon. 2012. "Making Quality Care Affordable for the Poor: Faith-Inspired Health Facilities in Burkina Faso." In Jill Olivier and Quentin Wodon (eds) *Mapping, Cost, and Reach to the Poor of Faith-Inspired Health Care Providers in Sub-Saharan Africa: Strengthening the Evidence for Faith-Inspired Health Engagement in Africa, Volume 3.* Washington, DC: The World Bank, pp 102–120.

Gerring, John. 2007. *Case Study Research: Principles and Practices.* Cambridge: Cambridge University Press.

Giusti, Daniele. no date. *Between a Rock and a Hard Place: The Commitment of CHSs to PHC.* Kampala, Uganda: Uganda Catholic Medical Bureau.

Gómez, Oscar A. and Des Gaspar. 2012. *Human Security A Thematic Guidance Note for Regional and National Human Development Report Teams.* United Nations Development Programme, Human Development Report Office. New York, NY: United Nations.

Government of Uganda. 2002. "Uganda Population and Housing Census, 2002." Available at: www.ubos.org/onlinefiles/uploads/ubos/census_tabulations/centableB7.pdf#page=1&zoom=auto,-73,798

Gros, Jean-Germain. 2016. *Healthcare Policy in Africa: Institutions and Politics from Colonialism to the Present*. Lanham, MD: Rowman & Littlefield.

Gunderson, Gary and James R. Cochrane. 2012. "Building on the Strengths of People Who Congregate." In Jill Olivier and Quentin Wodon (eds) *The Role of Faith-Inspired Health Care Providers in Sub-Saharan Africa and Public–Private Partnerships: Strengthening the Evidence for Faith-Inspired Health Engagement in Africa, Volume 1*. Washington, DC: The World Bank, pp 29–48.

Guttmacher Institute. 2013a. "Abortion in Uganda." January. Available at: www.guttmacher.org/pubs/FB-Abortion-in-Uganda.html#10

Guttmacher Institute. 2013b. "Fact Sheet on Contraception and Unintended Pregnancy in Uganda." September, www.guttmacher. org, accessed July 2017.

Guttmacher Institute. 2015. "Facts on Abortion in Africa 2015." Available at: www.guttmacher.org/pubs/IB_AWW-Africa.pdf, (accessed July 2017).

Guttmacher Institute. 2017a. "Abortion and Postabortion Care in Uganda." Fact sheet, February. Available at: www.guttmacher.org/ fact-sheet/abortion-and-postabortion-care-uganda (accessed July 2017).

Guttmacher Institute. 2017b. "Access to Safe Abortion Care in Ethiopia has Improved Following Expansion of Services." January 13. Available at: www.guttmacher.org (accessed July 2017).

Hacker, Jacob. 2006. *The Great Risk Shift*. New York, NY: Oxford University Press.

Hambuba, Carlyn. 2013. "The Maputo Protocol on Women's Rights in Africa: Is It an Answer to the Injustices That African Women Experience?" Blog entry, November 10.

Hamlin Hospital. 2017. "Hamlin Fistula Ethiopia." Available at: www. hamlin.org (accessed July 2017).

Hankivsky, Olena. 2012. *Health Inequities in Canada: Intersectional Frameworks and Practices*. Vancouver, BC: UBC Press.

Harron, Connor. 2015. "Challenges for Recovery in the Face of a Sustained HIV/AIDS Crisis and Structural Mismanagement: Lessons from Swaziland." Paper presented at the Annual Meeting of the International Studies Association (West), Pasadena, CA.

Hassner, Ron. 2009, 2012. *War on Sacred Grounds*. Ithaca, NY: Cornell University Press.

Hassner, Ron. 2016. *Religion on the Battlefield*. Ithaca, NY: Cornell University Press.

Hatzopoulos, Pavlos and Fabio Petito. 2003. "The Return from Exile: An Introduction." In Pavlos Hatzopoulos and Fabio Petito (eds) *Religion in International Relations: The Return from Exile*. New York, NY: Palgrave Macmillan.

Haussman, Melissa. 2005. *Abortion Politics in North America*. Boulder, CO: Lynne Rienner.

Haynes, Jeffrey. 2013. *An Introduction to International Relations and Religion* (2nd edn). Harlow: Pearson.

Henriksen, Sarita Monjane. 2014. "Identity and Plurilinguism in Africa—The case of Mozambique." *Acta Semiótica et Lingvistica* 19(2): 16–20.

Hinnells, John R. 2010. "Why Study Religions?" In John R. Hinnells (ed) *The Routledge Companion to the Study of Religion* (2nd edn). New York, NY: Routledge, pp 5–20.

Hodgett, Susan, and David Clark. 2011. "Capabilities, Well-Being and Multiculturalism: A New Framework for Guiding Policy." *International Journal of Canadian Studies* 44: 163–184.

Hodgett, Susan, and Peter Doran. 2018. "Societal Wellbeing – Catalyst for Systems and Social Change in Northern Ireland?" In Ian Bache and Karen Scott (eds). *The Politics of Wellbeing: Theory, Policy and Practice*. New York, NY: Palgrave.

Hoffman, Henryk. 2010. "The Methodology of Classical Religious Studies: A. N. Krasnikov's Evaluation." *Anthropos* 105(1): 233–238.

Holy Bible. 2004. *Holy Bible*, New Living Translation. Carol Stream, IL: Tyndale House Foundation.

Hönke, Jana and Christian R. Thauer. 2014. "Multinational Corporations and Service Provision in Sub-Saharan Africa: Legitimacy and Institutionalization Matter." Governance: An International Journal of Policy, Administration, and Institutions 27(4): 697–716. Available at: www.c-changeprogram.org/sites/default/files/PHDP-Mozambique-Report-FINAL_0.pdf

Huang, Chin-Hao and Patrick James. 2014. "Blue, Green or Aquamarine? Taiwan and the Status Quo Preference in Cross-Strait Relations." China Quarterly 219: 670–692.

Huber, Machteld, J. André Knottnerus, Lawrence Green, Henriëtte van der Horst, Alejandro R Jadad, Daan Kromhout, Brian Leonard, Kate Lorig, Maria Isabel Loureiro, Jos W M van der Meer, Paul Schnabel, Richard Smith, Chris van Weel, Henk Smid. 2011. "How Should We Define Health?" *British Medical Journal* 343: 1–3.

Iannaccone, Laurence R. 1994. "Why Strict Churches Are Strong." *American Journal of Sociology* 99: 1180–1211.

Iannaccone, Laurence R. 1995. "Voodoo Economics? Reviewing the Rational Choice Approach to Religion." *Journal for the Scientific Study of Religion* 34: 76–89.

Iannaccone, Laurence R., Rodney Stark, and Roger Finke. 1998. "Rationality and the 'Religious Mind'." *Economic Inquiry* 36: 373–389.

International Justice Resource Center. 2016. "Human Rights Commission Launches Campaign to Decriminalize Abortion." February 2. Available at: www.ijrcenter.org (accessed July 2017).

Inter-Parliamentary Union. 2016. "Homepage." www.ipu.org/english/home.htm

Iqbal, Zaryab. 2010. *War and the Health of Nations*. Palo Alto, CA: Stanford University Press.

Jacobsson, Lars. 2002. "Traditional Treatment of Mental and Psychosomatic Disorders in Ethiopia." *International Congress Series*, vol 1241, Elsevier.

Jagwe-Wadda, Gabriel, Ann M. Moore and Vanessa Woog. 2006. "Abortion Morbidity in Uganda: Evidence from Two Communities." Occasional Report No. 26, pp 1–58. Accessed at www.guttmacher.org/sites/default/files/report_pdf/or26.pdf, November 11, 2018.

Johnston, Douglas and Cynthia Sampson (eds). 1995. *Religion, the Missing Dimension of Statecraft*. Oxford: Oxford University Press.

Kabayambi, Joan. 2013. "Revisiting the Policy on Traditional Birth Attendants." May 10. Available at: www.allafrica.com (accessed February 15, 2016).

Kafeero, Stephen and Sandra Janet Birungi. 2014. "Uganda Tops Child Dependency Ratio in Region-UN." *Uganda Monitor*, August 15.

Kagimu, Magid. 2012. *The Interrelationship between Religiosity and HIV Infections in Uganda: A Community Case Study*. PhD, Public Health. Kampala: Makerere University.

Kagimu, Magid, David Guwatudde, Charles Rwabukwali, Sarah Kaye, Yusuf Walakira, and Dick Ainomugisha. 2011. "Inter-Religious Cooperation for HIV Prevention in Uganda: A Study Among Muslim and Christian Youth in Wakiso District." *Religions* 2: 707–728.

Kagimu, Magid, David Guwatudde, Charles Rwabukwali, Sarah Kaye, Yusuf Walakira, and Dick Ainomugisha. 2012a. "Religiosity for HIV Prevention in Uganda: A Case Study Among Christian Youth in Wakiso District." *African Health Sciences* 12: 17–25.

Kagimu, Magid, David Guwatudde, Charles Rwabukwali, Sarah Kaye, Yusuf Walakira, and Dick Ainomugisha. 2012b. "Religiosity for HIV Prevention in Uganda: A Case Study Among Muslim Youth in Wakiso District." *African Health Sciences* 12: 282–290.

References

Kagimu, Magid, Sarah Kaye, Dick Ainomugisha, I. Lutalo, Yusuf Walakira, David Guwatudde, and Charles Rwabukwali. 2012c. "Evidence-Based Monitoring and Evaluation of the Faith-Based Approach to HIV Prevention Among Christian and Muslim Youth in Wakiso District in Uganda." *African Health Sciences* 12: 119–128.

Kagimu, Magid, Sarah Kaye, Yusuf Walakira, David Guwatudde, Charles Rwabukwali, and Dick Ainomugisha. 2012d. "The Role of Religiosity in HIV Prevention in Uganda: A Case-Control Study Among Muslims and Christian Youth in Wakiso District." *World Journal of AIDS* 2: 286–293.

Kagimu, Magid, David Guwatudde, Charles Rwabukwali, Sarah Kaye, Yusuf Walakira, and Dick Ainomugisha. 2013. "Religiosity for Promotion of Behaviors Likely to Reduce New HIV Infections in Uganda: A Study Among Muslim Youth in Wakiso District." *Journal of Religion and Health* 52: 1211–1227.

Kamatenesi-Mugisha, Maud and Hannington Oryem-Origa. 2005. "Traditional Herbal Remedies Used in the Management of Sexual Impotence and Erectile Dysfunction in Western Uganda." *African Health Sciences* 5(1): 40–49. Available at: www.ncbi.nlm.nih.gov/pmc/articles/PMC1831906/

Karam, Azza. 2012. "The United Nations Population Fund's Legacy: Engaging Faith-Based Organizations as Cultural Agents of Change for the MDGs." In Jill Olivier and Quentin Wodon (eds) *The Role of Faith-Inspired Health Care Providers in Sub-Saharan Africa and Public–Private Partnerships: Strengthening the Evidence for Faith-Inspired Health Engagement in Africa, Volume 1*. Washington, DC: The World Bank, pp 140–149.

Kaufman, Stuart J. 2017. "Symbolic Politics as International Relations Theory." *Oxford Research Encyclopedia, Politics*. http://oxfordre.com/politics/view/10.1093/acrefore/9780190228637.001.0001/acrefore-9780190228637-e-323

Kaufmann, Judith R. and Harley Feldbaum. 2009. "Diplomacy and the Polio Immunization Boycott in Northern Nigeria." *Health affairs* 28(4): 1091–1101.

King, Gary, and Christopher J.L. Murray. 2002. "Rethinking Human Security." *Political Science Quarterly* 116: 585–610.

Kinsman, John. 2010. *AIDS Policy in Uganda: Evidence, Ideology, and the Making of an African Success Story*. New York, NY: Palgrave Macmillan.

Kisangani, Emizet. 1997. *Zaire after Mobutu: A Case of Humanitarian Emergency*. Helsinki: United Nations.

Kisangani, Emizet. 2012. *Civil Wars in the Democratic Republic of Congo, 1960–2010*. Boulder, CO: Lynne Rienner Publishers.

209

Koenig, Sybelle and Frazier Goodwin. 2011. "Health Spending in Mozambique: The Impact of Current Aid Structures and Aid Effectiveness." *EU Health ODA and Aid Effectiveness, Country Briefing 4*, Action for Global Health, the German Foundation for World Population.

Krishnamani, Pavitra. 2015a. "Global Goals for our Generation." *The New Physician* 64(6): 2.

Krishnamani, Pavitra. 2015b. "Where the Waiting Rooms Have No Chairs." *The New Physician* 64(6): 22–25.

Kumar, P. Pratap. 2006. "Religious Pluralism and Religion Education in South Africa." *Method & Theory in the Study of Religion* 18(3): 273–293.

Kumie, Abera and Year II Medical Students. 2005/2006. *Latrine Use and Cultural Values in Rural Population*. Addis Ababa: Addis Ababa University, School of Public Health.

Leslau, Wolf. 1961. "The Names of the Weekdays in Ethiopic." *Journal of Semitic Studies* 6: 62.

Linke, Andrew M., John O'Loughlin, J. Terrence McCabe, Jaroslav Tir, and Frank D.W. Witmer. 2015. "Rainfall Variability and Violence in Rural Kenya: Investigating the Effects of Drought and the Role of Institutions with Survey Data." *Global Environmental Change* 34: 35–47.

Linke, Andrew M., Frank D.W. Witmer, John O'Loughlin, J. Terrence McCabe, and Jaroslav Tir. forthcoming. "Drought, Local Institutional Contexts, and Support for Violence in Kenya." *Journal of Conflict Resolution*.

Lloyd, Robert. 2011. "Countries at the Crossroads 2011: Mozambique." Freedom House, Washington, DC. Available at: www.freedomhouse. org/report/countries-crossroads/2011/mozambique#.U-80NWMn_78

Lodhi, Abdulaziz Y. 1993. "The Language Situation in Africa Today." *Nordic Journal of African Studies* 2(1): 79–86.

Lugalambi, George W., Peter G. Mwesige, and Hendrik Bussiek. 2010. *Uganda: A Survey by the Africa Governance Monitoring and Advocacy Project (AfriMAP), Open Society Initiative for East Africa (OSIEA) and Open Society Media Program (OSMP)*. Johannesburg, South Africa: Open Society Initiative for East Africa.

Maioni, Antonia. 1998. *Parting at the Crossroads: The Emergence of Health Insurance in the United States and Canada*. New Jersey, NJ: Princeton University Press.

Make Every Woman Count. 2016. "African Women's Decade 2010–2020: Mid-Term Review." Available at: www.makeeverywomancount.org/index.php/african-womens-decade/african-womens-decade-2010-2020-annual-report/9804-african-women-s-decade-2010-2020-mid-term-review-2015-2016 (accessed July 22, 2017).

Malley, Brian E. 2013. "Toward an Engaged Religious Studies." In Scott S. Elliott (ed). *Reinventing Religious Studies: Key Writings in the History of a Discipline*. Bristol, CT: Acumen, pp 218–220.

"Maputo Protocol turns 15! A call for States to ratify and implement the Protocol-moving from rhetoric to action." July 11, 2018. Centre for Human Rights, Faculty of Law, University of Pretoria, accessed at www.chr.up.ac.za November 11, 2018.

Manning, Carrie L. 2002. *The Politics of Peace in Mozambique: Post-Conflict Democratization, 1992–2000*. Westport, CT: Greenwood Publishing Group.

Markakis, John. 2011. *Ethiopia: The Last Two Frontiers*. New York, NY: James Currey.

Martin, William G. 2011. "The Rise of African Studies (USA) and the Transnational Study of Africa." *African Studies Review* 54(1): 59–83.

Masinde, Andrew. 2013. "Despite the Ban, FGM Still Rears Its Ugly Head in Uganda." *New Vision*, February 5. Available at: www.newvision.co.ug (accessed July 22, 2017).

Mathers, Kathryn. 2016. "Framed: Representations of the Western Imagination of Africa." *USC Public Diplomacy Magazine* 15(Winter): 19–25.

Mbiti, John S. 1969. *African Religions & Philosophy*. London: Heinemann.

MDG Global Database. 2015a. "Ethiopia." August. Available at: http://mdgs.un.org/unsd/mdg/Data.aspx (accessed June 29, 2017).

MDG Global Database. 2015b. "Mozambique." August. Available at: http://mdgs.un.org/unsd/mdg/Data.aspx (accessed June 29, 2017).

MDG Global Database. 2015c. "Uganda." August. Available at: http://mdgs.un.org/unsd/mdg/Data.aspx (accessed June 29, 2017).

Meier, Barbara and Ames S. Steinforth (eds). 2014. *Spirits in Politics: Uncertainties of Power and Healing in African Societies*. Frankfurt and New York, NY: Campus Verlag.

Menkhaus, Ken. 2014. "State Collapse and Local Response in Somalia." In Ingo Trauschweizer and Steven M. Miner (eds) *Failed States and Fragile Societies: A New World Disorder?* Athens, OH: Ohio University Press, pp 142–149.

Mhame, Paulo Peter, Kofi Busia, and M.J. Ossy. 2010. "Clinical Practices of African Traditional Medicine." In World Health Organization (ed) *African Health Monitor 13*. Geneva, Switzerland: World Health Organization.

Mikkonen, Juha and Dennis Raphael. 2010. *Social Determinants of Health: The Canadian Facts*. Toronto: York University School of Health Policy and Management.

Ministry of Health, Government of Uganda. 2010. *Health Sector Strategic Plan III: 2010–15*. Kampala: Government of Uganda.

Ministry of Health, Government of Uganda. 2015. *National Village Health Teams (VHT) Assessment in Uganda*. Kampala: Government of Uganda.

Ministry of Planning and Development, Government of Mozambique. 2010. "Report on the Millennium Development Goals: Mozambique 2010." Available at: www.mz.undp.org/content/mozambique/en/home/library/mdg/-mozambique-mdg-report-2010/

Moftah, Lora. 2014. "Mozambique Legalizes Abortion: President Signs Law Seeking to Curb High Maternal Mortality Rate." *International Business Times*, December 19.

Molle, Mitika, Yemane Berhane, and Bernt Lindtjørn. 2008. "Traditional Values of Virginity and Sexual Behaviour in Rural Ethiopian Youth: Results from a Cross-Sectional Study." BMC Public Health 8: 9. Available at: www.ncbi.nlm.nih.gov/pmc/articles/PMC2254614/

Mortada, Dalia. 2014. "Ethiopia's Game-Changing Abortion Law." *Irin News*, August 8. Available at: www.irinnews.org (accessed July 2017).

Mossialos, Elias, Govin Permanand, Rita Baeten, and Tamara Hervey (eds). 2010. *Health Systems Governance in Europe: The Role of European Law and Policy*. Cambridge: Cambridge University Press.

Moyser, George. 2010. "Religion and Politics." In John R. Hinnells (ed) *The Routledge Companion to the Study of Religion* (2nd edn). New York, NY: Routledge, pp 445–460.

Muhirwe, Lorna B. 2012. "Approaches for Integrating Primary Health Care in Reproductive Health Programs in Uganda." In Jill Olivier and Quentin Wodon (eds) *The Role of Faith-Inspired Health Care Providers in Sub-Saharan Africa and Public–Private Partnerships: Strengthening the Evidence for Faith-Inspired Health Engagement in Africa, Volume 1*. Washington, DC: The World Bank, pp 134–142.

Mutebi, Brian. 2016. "Female Circumcision: Uganda Still Has a Long Way to Zero Tolerance." *Daily Monitor*, February 6.

Najjumba, Innocent Mulindwa, James Habyarimana and Charles Lwanga Bunjo. 2013. *Improved Learning in Uganda, Volume III: School-Based Management: Policy and Functionality*. Washington, DC: The World Bank.

Natala, Venrick. 2006. "Poverty and Public Health Care as an Impediment to Development in Uganda." In Syed A.H. Abidi (ed) *Peace in Uganda: The Role of the Civil Society*. Kampala: ABTO, pp 137–147.

Neusner, Jacob. 2013. "Religious Studies: The Next Vocation." In Scott S. Elliott (ed) *Reinventing Religious Studies: Key Writings in the History of a Discipline*. Bristol, CT: Acumen, pp 38–42.

New Vision: Uganda's Leading Daily. 2015. "Parliament, IPU Sign MoU on Women and Children's Health." September 16.

Njihia, C., C. Ambasa, W. Parker, and S. Rogers. 2012. *Perspectives of People Living with HIV on HIV Prevention: Opportunities and Challenges for Strengthening the Response in Mozambique*. Washington, DC: C-Change/FHI 360.

Norris, Pippa and Ronald Inglehart. 2004. *Sacred and Secular: Religion and Politics Worldwide*. Cambridge: Cambridge University Press.

Obinna, Elijah. 2012. "'Life is Superior to Wealth?' Indigenous Healers in an African Community, Amasiri, Nigeria." In Afe Adogame, Ezra Chitando, and Bolaji Bateye (eds) *African Traditions in the Study of Religion in Africa: Emerging Trends, Indigenous Spirituality and the Interface with Other World Religions*. Burlington, VT: Ashgate, pp 135–147.

Olivier, Jill and Beverly Haddad. 2012. "Christian Organizations' Place in Multisectoral HIV/AIDS Response: Kenya, Malawi and the Democratic Republic of Congo." In Jill Olivier and Quentin Wodon (eds) *The Role of Faith-Inspired Health Care Providers in Sub-Saharan Africa and Public–Private Partnerships: Strengthening the Evidence for Faith-Inspired Health Engagement in Africa, Volume 1*. Washington, DC: The World Bank, pp 167–182.

Olivier, Jill and Quentin Wodon. 2012a. "Mapping Cost, and Reach to the Poor of Faith-Inspired Health Care Providers in Sub-Saharan Africa: A Brief Overview." In Jill Olivier and Quentin Wodon (eds) *Mapping, Cost, and Reach to the Poor of Faith-Inspired Health Care Providers in Sub-Saharan Africa: Strengthening the Evidence for Faith-Inspired Health Engagement in Africa, Volume 3*. Washington, DC: The World Bank, pp 1–6.

Olivier, Jill and Quentin Wodon. 2012b. "Layers of Evidence: Discourses and Typologies of Faith-Inspired Community Responses to HIV/AIDS in Africa." In Jill Olivier and Quentin Wodon (eds) *Mapping, Cost, and Reach to the Poor of Faith-Inspired Health Care Providers in Sub-Saharan Africa: Strengthening the Evidence for Faith-Inspired Health Engagement in Africa, Volume 3*. Washington, DC: The World Bank, pp 25–51.

Olivier, Jill and Quentin Wodon. 2012c. "Faith-Inspired Health Care Providers in Sub-Saharan Africa and Public Private Partnerships: A Brief Overview." In Jill Olivier and Quentin Wodon (eds) *The Role of Faith-Inspired Health Care Providers in Sub-Saharan Africa and Public–Private Partnerships: Strengthening the Evidence for Faith-Inspired Health Engagement in Africa, Volume 1*. Washington, DC: The World Bank, pp 1–10.

Olivier, Jill and Quentin Wodon. 2012d. "Market Share of Faith-Inspired Health Care Providers in Africa: Comparing Facilities and Multi-Purpose Integrated Household Survey Data." In Jill Olivier and Quentin Wodon (eds) *The Role of Faith-Inspired Health Care Providers in Sub-Saharan Africa and Public–Private Partnerships: Strengthening the Evidence for Faith-Inspired Health Engagement in Africa, Volume 1*. Washington, DC: The World Bank, pp 11–26.

Olivier, Jill and Quentin Wodon. 2012e. "Increased Funding for AIDS-Engaged (Faith-Based) Civil Society Organizations in Africa?" In Jill Olivier and Quentin Wodon (eds) *The Role of Faith-Inspired Health Care Providers in Sub-Saharan Africa and Public–Private Partnerships: Strengthening the Evidence for Faith-Inspired Health Engagement in Africa, Volume 1*. Washington, DC: The World Bank, pp 143–166.

Olivier, Jill and Quentin Wodon. 2012f. "The Comparative Nature of Faith-Inspired Health Care Provision in Sub-Saharan Africa: A Brief Overview." In Jill Olivier and Quentin Wodon (eds) *The Comparative Nature of Faith-Inspired Health Care Provision in Sub-Saharan Africa: Strengthening the Evidence for Faith-Inspired Health Engagement in Africa, Volume 2*. Washington, DC: The World Bank, pp 1–5.

Olivier, Jill and Quentin Wodon (eds). 2012g. *The Role of Faith-Inspired Health Care Providers in Sub-Saharan Africa and Public–Private Partnerships: Strengthening the Evidence for Faith-Inspired Health Engagement in Africa, Volume 1*. Washington, DC: The World Bank.

Olivier, Jill and Quentin Wodon (eds). 2012h. *The Comparative Nature of Faith-Inspired Health Care Provision in Sub-Saharan Africa: Strengthening the Evidence for Faith-Inspired Health Engagement in Africa, Volume 2*. Washington, DC: The World Bank.

Olivier, Jill and Quentin Wodon (eds). 2012i. *Mapping, Cost, and Reach to the Poor of Faith-Inspired Health Care Providers in Sub-Saharan Africa: Strengthening the Evidence for Faith-Inspired Health Engagement in Africa, Volume 3*. Washington, DC: The World Bank.

Olivier, Jill, Clarence Tsimpo, and Quentin Wodon. 2012a. "Do Faith-Inspired Health Care Providers in Africa Reach the Poor More Than Other Providers?" In Jill Olivier and Quentin Wodon (eds) *Mapping, Cost, and Reach to the Poor of Faith-Inspired Health Care Providers in Sub-Saharan Africa: Strengthening the Evidence for Faith-Inspired Health Engagement in Africa, Volume 3*. Washington, DC: The World Bank, pp 7–24.

Olivier, Jill, Clarence Tsimpo, and Quentin Wodon. 2012b. "Satisfaction with Faith-Inspired Health Care Services in Africa: Review and Evidence from Household Surveys." In Jill Olivier and Quentin Wodon (eds) *The Role of Faith-Inspired Health Care Providers in Sub-Saharan Africa and Public–Private Partnerships: Strengthening the Evidence for Faith-Inspired Health Engagement in Africa, Volume 1*. Washington, DC: The World Bank, pp 6–28.

Olivier, Jill, James R. Cochrane, and Steven de Gruchy. 2012c. "Mapping Religious Community Health Assets and Initiatives: Lessons from Zambia and Lesotho." In Jill Olivier and Quentin Wodon (eds) *Mapping, Cost, and Reach to the Poor of Faith-Inspired Health Care Providers in Sub-Saharan Africa: Strengthening the Evidence for Faith-Inspired Health Engagement in Africa, Volume 3*. Washington, DC: The World Bank, pp 52–61.

Olivier, Jill, Mari Shojo, and Quentin Wodon. 2012d. "Faith-Inspired Health Care Provision in Ghana: Market Share, Reach to the Poor, and Performance." In Jill Olivier and Quentin Wodon (eds) *The Role of Faith-Inspired Health Care Providers in Sub-Saharan Africa and Public–Private Partnerships: Strengthening the Evidence for Faith-Inspired Health Engagement in Africa, Volume 1*. Washington, DC: The World Bank, pp 118–133.

Olson, Laura Katz. 2010. *The Politics of Medicaid*. New York, NY: Columbia University Press.

Olupona, Jacob K. 2004 "Owner of the Day and Regulator of the Universe: Ifa Divination and Healing Among the Yoruba of South-Western Nigeria." In Michael Winkelman and Philip M. Peeks (eds). *Divination and Healing: Potent Vision*. Tucson, AZ: University of Arizona Press, pp. 103-117.

Orach, Sam Orochi. no date. "Is Religion Relevant in Health Care in Africa in the 21st century? The Uganda Experience." Available at: https://berkleycenter.georgetown.edu/publications/is-religion-relevant-in-health-care-in-africa-in-the-21st-century-the-uganda-experience

Organization of African Unity. 2001. "African Summit on HIV/AIDS, Tuberculosis and Other Related Infectious Diseases." Abuja, Nigeria, April 24–27. Available at: www.un.org/ga/aids/pdf/abuja_declaration.pdf

Pallant, Dean. 2012. "Global Health Provision for Development: The Salvation Army's Experience." In Jill Olivier and Quentin Wodon (eds) *The Role of Faith-Inspired Health Care Providers in Sub-Saharan Africa and Public–Private Partnerships: Strengthening the Evidence for Faith-Inspired Health Engagement in Africa, Volume 1*. Washington, DC: The World Bank, pp 89–100.

Paris, Roland. 2001. "Human Security: Paradigm Shift or Hot Air?" *International Security* 26: 87–102.

Parkhurst, Justin O. 2002. "The Ugandan Success Story? Evidence and Claims of HIV-1 Prevention." *The Lancet* 360: 78–80.

Periago, Mirta Roses. 2012. "Human Security and Public Health." *Pan American Journal of Public Health/Revista Panamericana de Salud Pública* 31: 355–358.

Pew Research Center. 2010. *Tolerance and Tension: Islam and Christianity in Sub-Saharan Africa*. Available at: www.pewforum.org/2010/04/15/executive-summary-islam-and-christianity-in-sub-saharan-africa/

Pew Research Center. 2011. "Religion & Public Life, Christian Population as Percentages of Total Population." December 19. Available at: www.pewforum.org/2011/12/19/table-christian-population-as-percentages-of-total-population-by-country/

Pfeiffer, James. 2005. "Commodity Fetichismo, the Holy Spirit, and the Turn to Pentecostal and African Independent Churches in Central Mozambique." *Culture, Medicine and Psychiatry* 29 (3): 255–283. Available at: http://link.springer.com/article/10.1007%2Fs11013-005-9168-3

Pfeiffer, James. 2011. "Pentecostalism and AIDS Treatment in Mozambique: Creating New Approaches to HIV Prevention Through Anti-Retroviral Therapy." *Global Public Health* 6(Supplement 2): S163–S173.

Pinkey, Robert. 2001. *The International Politics of East Africa*. Manchester: Manchester University Press.

Polity. 2010. "Polity IV Country Report 2010: Ethiopia." Available at: www.systemicpeace.org/polity/Ethiopia2010.pdf

PRI (Public Radio International). 2014. "How Ethiopia Solved Its Abortion Problem." September 8. Available at: www.pri.org (accessed July 2017).

Provost, Claire. 2014. "Ethiopia's Model Families Hailed as Agents of Social Transformation." *The Guardian*, January 9. Available at: www. theguardian.com (accessed July 2017).

Quinn, John James. 2016. *Global Geopolitical Power and African Political and Economic Institutions: When Elephants Fight*. Lanham, MD: Lexington Books.

Ragunathan, Muthuswamy, Hawi Tadesse, and Rebecca Tujuba. 2010. "A Cross-Sectional Study on the Perceptions and Practices of Modern and Traditional Health Practitioners About Traditional Medicine in Dembia District, North Western Ethiopia." *Pharmacognosy Magazine* 6(21): 19–25.

Ranger, T.O. 1988. "African Traditional Religion." In Peter Clarke and Stewart Sutherland (eds) *The World's Religions: The Study of Religion, Traditional and New Religion*. London: Routledge, pp 106–114.

Raphael, Dennis. 2009. "Social Determinants of Health: An Overview of Key Issues and Themes." In Dennis Raphael (ed) *Social Determinants of Health: Canadian Perspectives*. Toronto: Canadian Scholars' Press Inc, pp 2–19.

Raschke, Carl A. 2013. "The Future of Religious Studies: Moving Beyond the Mandate of the 1960s." In Scott S. Elliott (ed) *Reinventing Religious Studies: Key Writings in the History of a Discipline*. Bristol, CT: Acumen, pp 51–55.

Republic of Mozambique. December 18, 2013. *Report on the Millennium Development Goals, 2010*. Maputo: Republic of Mozambique. Accessed at.www.mz.undp.org, July 2017.

Richard, Fabienne, David Hercot, Charlemagne Ouédraogo, Thérèse Delvaux, Salif Samaké, Josefien van Olmen, Ghislaine Conombo, Rachel Hammonds, and Jan Vandemoortele. 2011. "Sub-Saharan Africa and the Health MDGs: The Need to Move Beyond the 'Quick Impact' Model." *Reproductive Health Matters* 19(38): 42–55.

Roudi-Fahimi, Farzaneh. 2004. *Islam and Family Planning*. Washington, DC: Population Reference Bureau.

Saltman, Richard, Reinhard Busse, and Josep Figueras. 2004. *Social Health Insurance Systems in Western Europe*. New York, NY: Open University Press.

Sama, Martyn and Vinh-Kim Nguyen (eds). 2008. *Governing Health Systems in Africa*. Dakar, Senegal: Codesria Press.

Sandal, Nukhet A. and Jonathan Fox. 2013. *Religion in International Relations Theory: Interactions and Possibilities*. London and New York, NY: Routledge.

Schäferhoff, Marco. 2014. "External Actors and the Provision of Public Health Services in Somalia." *Governance: An International Journal of Policy, Administration, and Institutions* 27(4): 675–695.

Schmid, Barbara, Elizabeth Thomas, Jill Olivier, and James Cochrane. 2008. *The Contribution of Religious Entities to Health in Sub-Saharan Africa*. Study Commissioned by B & M Gates Foundation, unpublished report. African Religious Health Assets Programme (ARHAP).Cape Town: University of Cape Town.

Segal, Robert A. 2010. "Theories of Religion." In John R. Hinnells (ed) *The Routledge Companion to the Study of Religion* (2nd edn). New York, NY: Routledge, pp 75–92.

Segal, Robert A. 2013. "Fending Off the Social Sciences." In Scott S. Elliott (ed) *Reinventing Religious Studies: Key Writings in the History of a Discipline*. Bristol, CT: Acumen, pp 86–90.

Sharma, Arvind. 2005. *Religious Studies and Comparative Methodology: The Case for Reciprocal Illumination*. Albany, NY: SUNY Press.

Sharma, Arvind. 2013. "The Academic Study of Religion: A Methodological Reflection." In Scott S. Elliott (ed) *Reinventing Religious Studies: Key Writings in the History of a Discipline*. Bristol, CT: Acumen, pp 83–85.

Sharpe, Eric J. 2010. "The Study of Religion in Historical Perspective." In John R. Hinnells (ed) *The Routledge Companion to the Study of Religion* (2nd edn). New York, NY: Routledge, pp 21–38.

Shiferaw, Solomon, Mark Spigt, Merjin Godefrooij, Yilma Melkamu, and Michael Tekie. 2013. "Why Do Women Prefer Home Births in Ethiopia?" *BMC Pregnancy and Childbirth* 13: 5.

Shinn, David H. and Thomas P. Ofcansky. 2004. *Historical Dictionary of Ethiopia* (new edn). Lanham, MD: The Scarecrow Press.

Shojo, Mari, Clarence Tsimpo, and Quentin Wood. 2012. "Satisfaction With and Reasons for Choosing Faith-Inspired Health Care Provision in Ghana." In Jill Olivier and Quentin Wodon (eds) *The Role of Faith-Inspired Health Care Providers in Sub-Saharan Africa and Public–Private Partnerships: Strengthening the Evidence for Faith-Inspired Health Engagement in Africa, Volume 1*. Washington, DC: The World Bank, pp 73–88.

Shuey, D. A., B. B. Babishangire, S. Omiat and H. Bagarukayo. 1999. "Increased Sexual Abstinence Among In-School Adolescents as a Result of School Health Education in Soroti District, Uganda." *Health Education Research* 14: 411–419.

Sidaway, James D. and Marcus Power. 1995. "Sociospatial Transformations in the 'Postsocialist' Periphery: The Case of Maputo, Mozambique." *Environment and Planning A* 27(9): 1463–1491.

Sigsworth, Romi and liezelle Kumalo. 2016. *Women, Peace and Security: Implementing the Maputo Protocol in Africa*. ISS Paper 295, July, pp 1–24. Dakar, Ethiopia, Kenya and South Africa: Institute for Security Studies.

Sim, Fiona and Martin McKee. 2011. *Issues in Public Health* (2nd edn). New York, NY: Open University Press.

Singh, Susheela, Elena Prada, Florence Mirembe and Charles Kiggundu. 2005. "The Incidence of Induced Abortion in Uganda," *International Family Planning Perspectives* 31(4): 183–192. Available at: www.guttmacher.org/journals/ipsrh/2005/12/incidence-induced-abortion-uganda

Siu, Godfrey E., and Susan R. Whyte. 2009. "Increasing Access to Health Education in Eastern Uganda: Rethinking the Role and Preparation of Volunteers." *Health Education Journal* 68: 83–93.

Slikkerveer, Leendert Jan. 1982. "Rural Health Development in Ethiopia: Problem of Utilization of Traditional Healers." *Social Science Medicine* 16: 1859–1872.

Starr, Paul. 1982. *The Social Transformation of American Medicine: The Rise of a Sovereign Profession and the Making of a Vast Industry*. New York, NY: Basic Books.

Sutherland, Stewart. 1988. "The Study of Religion and Religions." In Peter Clarke and Stewart Sutherland (eds). *The World's Religions: The Study of Religion, Traditional and New Religion*. London: Routledge, pp 29–40.

Suzuki, Mao. 2015. *When Human Rights Demands Change a Pharmaceutical Company's Decision in Relation to Access to Medicines: Process-Tracing Analysis of AIDS Drug "d4T."* Los Angeles, CA: University of Southern California.

Takemi, Keizo, Masamine Jimba, Sumie Ishii, Yasushi Katsuma and Yasuhide Nakamura. 2008a. "Human Security Approach for Global Health." *The Lancet* 372(9632): 13–14.

Takemi, Keizo, Masmine Jimba, Sumie Ishii, Yasushi Katsuma, and Yasuhide Nakamura. 2008b. "Global Health as a Human Security Challenge." Background paper for the Trilateral Commission 2008 Annual Meeting.

Tatalovich, Raymond. 1997. *The Politics of Abortion in the United States and Canada: A Comparative Study*. Armonk, NY: M.E. Sharpe.

Tilahun, Mesfin, Bezatu Mengistie, Gudina Egata, and Ayalu A. Reda. 2012. "Health Workers' Attitudes Toward Sexual and Reproductive Health Services for Unmarried Adolescents in Ethiopia." *Reproductive Health* 9: 19.

Toefy, Yoesrie. 2009. "HIV/AIDS, Religion and Spirituality." In Poul Rohleder, Leslie Swartz, Seth Kalichman and Leickness Chisamu Simbayi (eds) *HIV/AIDS in South Africa 25 Years On: Psychosocial Perspectives*, New York, NY: Springer.

Toft, Monica Duffy, Daniel Philpott, and Timothy Samuel Shah. 2011. *God's Century: Resurgent Religion and Global Politics*. New York, NY: W.W. Norton & Company.

Tolchinsky, Marina. 2013. *Faith-Based Organizations (FBOs) and Public Health in Sub-Saharan Africa*. Senior thesis, School of International Relations. Los Angeles, CA: University of Southern California.

TradingEconomics.com. no date. "Rural Population in Mozambique." Available at: www.tradingeconomics.com (accessed February 16, 2016).

Transparency International. 2013. "Corruption Perceptions Index." Available at: http://cpi.transparency.org/cpi2013/results/

Transparency International. 2014. "Corruption Perceptions Inde: Ethiopia." Available at: www.transparency.org/country#ETH

Trinitapoli, Jenny. 2006. "Religious Responses to AIDS in Sub-Saharan Africa: An Examination of Religious Congregations in Rural Malawi." *Review of Religious Research* 47(3): 253–270.

Trinitapoli, Jenny and Alexander Weinreb. 2012. *Religion and AIDS in Africa*. New York, NY: Oxford University Press.

Tronvoll, Kjetil and Tobias Hagmann (eds). 2011. *Contested Power in Ethiopia: Traditional Authorities and Multi-Party Elections* (vol 27). Boston, MA: Brill.

Tsimpo, Clarence and Quentin Wodon. 2012. "Differences in the Private Cost of Health Care between Providers and Satisfaction with Services: Results for Sub-Saharan Countries." In Jill Olivier and Quentin Wodon (eds) *Mapping, Cost, and Reach to the Poor of Faith-Inspired Health Care Providers in Sub-Saharan Africa: Strengthening the Evidence for Faith-Inspired Health Engagement in Africa, Volume 3*. Washington, DC: The World Bank, pp 76–90.

Tuohy, Carolyn Hughes. 1999. *Accidental Logics: The Dynamics of Change in the Health-Care Arena in the United States, Britain and Canada*. New York, NY: Oxford University Press.

Turner, Harold W. 1981. "The Way Forward in the Religious Study of African Primal Religions." *Journal of Religion in Africa* 12(1): 1–15.

Turner, Harold W. 1988. "Africa." In Peter Clarke and Stewart Sutherland (eds). *The World's Religions: The Study of Religion, Traditional and New Religion*. London: Routledge, pp 187–194.

Uganda Ministry of Finance, Development and Economic Planning. 2013. "Millennium Development Goals Report for Uganda 2013." September. Available at: www.ug.undp.org/content/dam/uganda/docs/UNDPUg-2013MDGProgress%20Report-Oct%202013.pdf

Uganda Village Project. 2015. "Village Health Teams." Available at: www.ugandavillageproject.org/

UN. 1986. "Prevalence of Induced Abortion in Uganda." UN Population Division, Department of Social and Economic Affairs.

UN. 2013. "Mozambique." Human Development Report. Available at: www.hdr.undp.org/sites/default/files/Country-Profiles/MOZ.pdf

UN. 2015a. "The Millennium Development Goals Report."

UN. 2015b. "Trends in Contraceptive Use Worldwide." Department of Economic and Social Affairs, Population Division.

UNAIDS (Joint United Nations Programme on HIV and AIDS). 2013. "New HIV Infections Among Children Have Been Reduced by 50% or More in 7 Countries in Sub-Saharan Africa." Geneva. Available at: www.unaids.org (accessed July 2017).

UNAIDS. 2017. "The Living Legacy of the Global Plan." Available at: www.unaids.org (accessed July 2017).

UNDP (United Nations Development Programme). 2016. "Improving Maternal Health: Where do We Stand?" Available at: www.undp.org (accessed February 15, 2016).

UNFPA (United Nations Population Fund). 2010. "Sexual and Reproductive Health for All." September.

UNFPA. 2011. "Causes and Consequences of Population Growth in Mozambique." October 25. Available at: www.unfpa.org/news/causes-and-consequences-population-growth-mozambique

UNICEF (United Nations Children's Fund). no date. "Goal: Improve Maternal Health." Available at: www.unicef.org/mdg/maternal.html (accessed February 17, 2016).

United Nations Development Programme. 1994. *Human Development Report 1994*. New York, NY: Oxford University Press.

United Nations Economic Commission for Africa. 2015. "Assessing progress in Africa toward the millennium development goals." Available at: www.uneca.org/publications/mdg-report-2015-assessing-progress-africa-toward-millennium-development-goals

UN NGLS (United Nations, Non-Governmental Liaison Service). 2010. "African Women's Decade (2010–2020) Officially Launched on International Day of Rural Women." November or December. Available at: https://genderlinks.org.za/programme-web-menu/publications/roadmap-to-equality-issue-12-november-2010-2010-11-09/ (accessed July 2017).

Unruh, Jon D., Nikolas C Heynen, and Peter Hossler. 2003. "The Political Ecology of Recovery from Armed Conflict: The Case of Landmines in Mozambique." Political Geography 22: 841–861.

Vernoff, Charles Elliott. 2013. "Naming the Game: A Question of the Field." In Scott S. Elliott (ed) Reinventing Religious Studies: Key Writings in the History of a Discipline. Bristol, CT: Acumen, pp 56–63.

Vogel, Ronald. 1993. Financing Health Care in Sub-Saharan Africa. Westport, CT: Greenwood Press.

Waage, Jeff, Rukmini Banerji, Oona Campbell, Ephraim Chirwa, Guy Collender, Veerle Dieltiens, Andrew Dorward, Peter Godfrey-Fausett, Piya Hanvoravongchai, Geeta Kingdon, Angela Little, Anne Mills, Kim Mulholland, Alywn Mwinga, Amy North, Walaiporn Patcharanarumol, Colin Poulton, Viroj Tangcharoensathien, and Elaine Unterhalter. 2010. "The Millennium Development Goals: A Cross-Sectoral Analysis and Principles for Goal Setting After 2015." The Lancet 376(9745): 991–1023.

Welle, Katharina. 2014. "Monitoring Performance or Performing Monitoring? Exploring the Power and Political Dynamics Underlying Monitoring the MDG for Rural Water in Ethiopia." Canadian Journal of Development Studies 35: 155–169.

Westerlund, David. 2006. African Indigenous Religions and Disease Causation: From Spiritual Beings to Living Humans. Boston, MA: Brill.

Wike, Richard and Katie Simmons. 2015. Health Care, Education Are Top Priorities in Sub-Saharan Africa. Washington, DC: Pew Research Center.

Wodon, Quentin, Minh Cong Nguyen, and Clarence Tsimpo. 2012. "Market Share of Faith-Inspired and Private Secular Health Care Providers in Africa: Comparing DHS and Multi-Purpose Integrated Surveys." In Jill Olivier and Quentin Wodon (eds) The Role of Faith-Inspired Health Care Providers in Sub-Saharan Africa and Public–Private Partnerships: Strengthening the Evidence for Faith-Inspired Health Engagement in Africa, Volume 1. Washington, DC: The World Bank, pp 27–40.

Woldemicael, Gebremariam and Eric Y. Tenkorang. 2010. "Women's Autonomy and Maternal Health-Seeking Behavior in Ethiopia." Maternal Child Health Journal 14: 988–998.

Wolffe, John. 2010. "Religious History." In John R. Hinnells (ed) *The Routledge Companion to the Study of Religion* (2nd edn). New York, NY: Routledge, pp 57–72.

World Bank: Ethiopia. 2016. "The World Bank in Ethiopia" Available at: www.worldbank.org/en/country/ethiopia (accessed October 13, 2016).

World Economic Forum. 2016. *The Global Gender Gap Report*. Geneva, Switzerland: World Economic Forum.

World Health Organization (WHO). no date. "Mozambique's Health System." Available at: www.who.int/countries/moz/areas/health_system/en/index1.html

World Health Organization. 2007. "Health Promotion: Achievements and Next Steps." Available at: www.who.int/countries/moz/areas/health_promotion/en/index2.html

World Health Organization. 2011. "The Abuja Declaration: Ten Years On, 2011." Available at: www.who.int/healthsystems/publications/Abuja10.pdf

World Health Organization. 2014. "Mozambique: Country Cooperation at a Glance." Available at: www.who.int/countryfocus/cooperation_strategy/ccsbrief_moz_en.pdf

World Health Organization. 2015. "World Health Statistics, 2015." Available at: www.who.int/gho/publications/world_health_statistics/2015/en/ (accessed July 2017).

World Health Organization. 2017. "Health Impact Assessment: The Social Determinants of Health." Available at: www.who.org (accessed July 2017).

World Health Organization, Regional Office for Africa. 2013. *WHO Country Cooperation Strategy, 2012–2015: Ethiopia*. Brazzaville, Republic of Congo: WHO, Regional Office for Africa.

World Health Organization, Regional Office for Africa. 2014. *The Health of the People: What Works—The African Regional Health Report 2014*. Brazzaville, Republic of Congo: World Health Organization.

World Trade Press. n.d. *Uganda: Society and Culture*. Petaluma, CA: World Trade Press.

World Vision. 2017. "Untying the Knot: 10 Worst Places for Child Marriage." Available at: www.worldvision.org (accessed July 2017).

World Vision Ethiopia. 2013. *Annual Report*. Addis Ababa: World Vision Ethiopia.

World Vision Ethiopia. 2014. *Quarterly Newsletter* 1(1). Available at: www.wvi.org/sites/default/files/Quarterly%20Newsletter%20final-for%20web.pdf

Yirga, Wondimu Shanko; Nega Assefa Kassa, Mengistu Welday, Gebremichael, and Arja R. Aro. 2012. "Female Genital Mutilation: Prevalence, Perceptions and Effect on Women's Health in Kersa District of Ethiopia." *International Journal of Women's Health* 4: 45–54.

York, Geoffrey. 2017. "Trudeau Government Unveils Reproductive Health Projects," *The Globe and Mail*, July 11.

Index

NOTE: page numbers in *italic type* refer to tables.

in Mozambique 113, 181
in Uganda 79
child mortality 4, 35, *37*, 76, 111,
139, 161–2, 178, 181
child sacrifice 68
cholera 103
Christian evangelism 2
Christian Workers Union for Health
Care in Ethiopia 163
Christians/Christianity
in Ethiopia 121
religiosity and HIV *56*
in Uganda *61*
see also Anglicans; Catholic Church;
Catholics
Church of Uganda (Anglican) 52
Citropsis articulata 65
civil society 183, 184
civil wars 10
clinics 91, 98, 105, 136, 141–2,
171–2
and government standards 143–4,
149
private 143
Cola acuminata 65
comparative advantage 29–30, 32
Consortium of Christian Relief and
Development Associations 117,
130, 131, 133, 136, 140–1, *144–5*
coordination of health care
provision 147
holistic approach 158
Constitutional Court of Uganda 71
consumers of health care 27
contraceptive use 4, *37*, 181
in Ethiopia 165, 175–6
in Mozambique 110, 112, 113, 114
in Uganda 74, 75–6, 78
Convention on the Elimination of all
Forms of Discrimination Against
Women 6, 7, 8, 160, 180
corruption
in Ethiopia 120
and the state 1
in Uganda 44, 63
Corruption Perceptions Index 44,
86–7, 120
curandeiros 97, 97n8, 99, 103
cost of services 103, 104, 105
"*curandeiro* problem" 104
earning income 105
and epilepsy 105

good and bad 106
importance in Mozambique 104
IURD view of 102
and mega-churches 109
and modern medicine 106
relationship between spiritual and
physical world 109
reliance on 106
use by Muslims 107
working with medical professionals
104–5, 108
see also traditional healers
Cyril, Saint, Patriarch of Alexandria
146

D

Department for International
Development 133
Department of Social and Economic
Affairs 76
depression 149
Dhlakama, Afonso 85–6
diseases 16
divination 27
Dollo Ado 160, 165
donor states 5–6

E

Eastern Orthodox Church (Ethiopia)
121
education
health 107
in Mozambique 107
in Uganda 44
Egerö, Bertil 84
elites, state 30
Emerging Churches (Igrejas
Emergentes) 96
empathy 128
epilepsy 105
Eritrea 120
Eritrean People's Liberation Front
120
Ethiopia
Battle of Adwa (1896) 119
child dependency ratio 176
child marriage 164
and Christianity 2
context 119–25
culture
conflict of religion and secular
West 133
homosexuality 133